Poor Families in America's Health Care Crisis examines the implications of the fragmented and two-tiered health insurance system in the United States for the health care access of low-income families. For a large fraction of Americans, their jobs do not provide health insurance or other benefits, and although government programs are available for children, adults without private health care coverage have few options. Detailed ethnographic and survey data from selected low-income neighborhoods in Boston, Chicago, and San Antonio document the lapses in medical coverage that poor families experience and reveal the extent of untreated medical conditions, delayed treatment, medical indebtedness, and irregular health care that women and children suffer as a result. Extensive poverty, the increasing proportion of minority households, and the growing dependence on insecure service-sector work all influence access to health care for families at the economic margin.

Ronald J. Angel, Ph.D., is Professor of Sociology at the University of Texas at Austin. With his wife, Jacqueline Angel, he is the author of *Painful Inheritance: Health and the New Generation of Fatherless Families* and *Who Will Care for Us? Aging and Long-Term Care in Multicultural America*. Professor Angel served as editor of the *Journal of Health and Social Behavior* from 1994 to 1997, and he has served on the editorial boards of numerous other journals. He has administered several large grants from NIA, NIMH, NICHD, and several private foundations.

Laura Lein, Ph.D., is Professor in the School of Social Work and the Department of Anthropology at the University of Texas at Austin. She received her doctorate in social anthropology from Harvard University in 1973. She is the author, with Kathryn Edin, of *Making Ends Meet: How Single Mothers Survive Welfare and Low-Wage Work*. She has published numerous articles, most recently in *Community, Work and Family, Violence Against Women*, and *Journal of Adolescent Research*.

Jane Henrici, Ph.D., is an Assistant Professor of Anthropology at the University of Memphis. She earned her doctorate from the University of Texas at Austin. She has published articles and chapters on development programs and their interaction with ethnicity and gender in Perú, as well as on social programs and their effects on poor women in the United States. With respect to the latter, she edited and contributed to a volume titled *Doing Without: Women and Work after Welfare Reform* (forthcoming). She is also the recipient of a Fulbright fellowship.

Poor Families in America's Health Care Crisis

RONALD J. ANGEL
The University of Texas at Austin

LAURA LEIN
The University of Texas at Austin

JANE HENRICI
University of Memphis

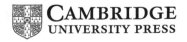
CAMBRIDGE
UNIVERSITY PRESS

CAMBRIDGE UNIVERSITY PRESS
Cambridge, New York, Melbourne, Madrid, Cape Town, Singapore, São Paulo

Cambridge University Press
40 West 20th Street, New York, NY 10011-4211, USA

www.cambridge.org
Information on this title: www.cambridge.org/9780521837743

First published 2006

Printed in the United States of America

A catalog record for this publication is available from the British Library.

Library of Congress Cataloging in Publication Data

Angel, Ronald.
Poor families in America's health care crisis / Ronald J. Angel, Laura Lein,
Jane Henrici.
  p. cm.
Includes bibliographical references and index.
ISBN 0-521-83774-X (hardcover) – ISBN 0-521-54676-1 (pbk.)
1. Poor – Medical care – United States – Finance. 2. Poor – Medical care –
Government policy – United States. 3. Medically uninsured persons – Medical care –
United States – Finance. 4. Insurance, Health – United States – Finance. 5. Health
services accessibility – Economic aspects – United States. 6. Equality – Health
aspects – United States. 7. Right to health care – United States. I. Title.
II. Laura Lein. III. Jane Henrici.
RA418.5.P6 A58 2006
362.5/82 22–pcc   2005028144

ISBN-13 978-0-521-83774-3 hardback
ISBN-10 0-521-83774-X hardback

ISBN-13 978-0-521-54676-8 paperback
ISBN-10 0-521-54676-1 paperback

Contents

Preface

The United States stands alone among developed nations in not providing publicly funded health care coverage to all citizens as a basic right. Rather than a universal and comprehensive tax-based system of care, our health care financing system consists of three main components: private insurance, consisting mostly of group plans sponsored by employers; Medicare for those over sixty-five; and a means-tested system of public coverage for poor children, the disabled, and low-income elderly individuals. Unfortunately, these three components are far from comprehensive. More than forty-five million Americans have no health care coverage of any sort, and millions more have episodic and inadequate coverage. As a consequence, the health care they receive is often inadequate, and their health is placed at risk. Although many of those without coverage receive charitable care or are seen at emergency rooms, they enjoy neither the continuity of care nor the high-quality care that fully insured Americans expect. As we demonstrate in this book, the lack of adequate health care coverage is part of a vicious cycle in which the poor face more serious risks to their health and receive less adequate preventive and acute care. Because minority Americans are more likely than majority Americans to be poor, this health and productivity penalty takes on an aspect of color. African Americans live shorter lives on average than white Americans do, and they suffer disproportionately from the preventable consequences of the diseases of poverty.

Because of the universally recognized fact that good health represents the foundation of a productive and happy life, in recent years the U.S. Congress has extended the health care safety net for poor children. Medicaid and the new State Children's Health Insurance Program (SCHIP) have extended medical coverage to nearly all children and teenagers in low-income families. Unfortunately, as we document in the following chapters, not all children who qualify on the basis of low family income are enrolled. For nondisabled adults under the age of sixty-five, no such programs exist. Pregnant women and those with serious disabilities, including HIV/AIDS, qualify for publicly funded health care, but adults who are not disabled or pregnant or those in families not receiving cash assistance have few options. Those who work in service-sector jobs are unlikely to be offered employer-sponsored group coverage that they can afford, and in the absence of universal health care they have no choice but to go into debt in the case of serious illness or simply do without care.

Conservatives and liberals approach health care financing and any potential reform of the current system from different perspectives. As is the case with other aspects of the welfare state, those approaches are based on different philosophies concerning individual responsibility and the role of the state in providing citizens with the necessities of a dignified and productive life. Health care, however, is different from other aspects of the welfare state, including cash assistance for the poor. Since the 1980s and 1990s, public disenchantment with cash assistance has led to a demand that the poor be forced to take more responsibility for their own welfare and not become wards of the state. As part of welfare reform, the entire apparatus of time limits, sanctions, and work requirements with which the states had experimented for a decade before the federal government made it the law of the land was put in place.

Even in this changed climate, with its rejection of long-term cash assistance, health care for the poor was recognized to be different. Welfare reform was intended to reduce the cash assistance rolls but not the Medicaid rolls. Medicaid use was, in fact, expected to increase, even though the unintended consequence of welfare reform was to reduce the Medicaid rolls at least in the short term. The expansion of public coverage for poor children represents a response to the new reality of medical care, one that increasingly affects working Americans. Since the 1970s, the cost of health care has grown at a rate far in excess of general inflation, and both employers and workers find that they must pay ever more for less coverage. Many employers have responded by requiring that their employees pay a larger part of the cost or by dropping their health plans altogether. Others have resorted to contingent and contract employment. As a result, a growing number of workers are not regular salaried employees and receive no retirement or health benefits from the enterprises to which they provide services. Today, a growing number of working Americans find themselves with no or inadequate health coverage. One can be a highly responsible working adult and find that one cannot obtain health care for one's family.

Health care coverage is not really an issue that belongs to the political right or left. Because a healthy population translates directly into a productive workforce, adequate health care directly serves the purposes of business in producing profits. Businesses that must compete globally with competitors in nations in which the workforce is covered by government-sponsored plans face a disadvantage if they must provide even tax-subsidized care to their workers. Universal access to adequate preventive and acute health care therefore benefits business interests as much as it does labor interests. Management and stockholders benefit as profits rise, and citizens in general benefit as healthy workers are able to pay taxes for Social Security and the rest of the middle-class welfare state.

In this book, we draw on newly collected survey and ethnographic data from three cities – Boston, Chicago, and San Antonio – to characterize the nature of the health care system and its consequences for low-income families. Given the reality of poverty and minority-group disadvantage in the United States, most of our sample is African American or Hispanic. Although the purpose of the study was to investigate the consequences of welfare reform for families and children in poverty, we learned much more about their lives, including how central issues of health are to the challenges they face. Much of what we document relates to the despair and humiliation, as well as the inadequate health care, that many families suffer because of their dependence on the means-tested and often stigmatizing system of health care financing for the poor.

We are clearly in favor of universal health care coverage in which all citizens, regardless of their ability to pay, receive basic preventive and acute care. As more working and even middle-class Americans find themselves without coverage that they can afford, the demand for a more equitable, rational, and comprehensive system will grow. Such a system will be expensive, and current debates revolve around the issue of how best to provide the best coverage to the greatest number of citizens at a sustainable cost. Whatever the ultimate route to universal coverage, however, we believe that it is eventually inevitable, both because of the indefensibility of the current highly inequitable and incomplete system and because of the unique and essentially public nature of health care.

The study that forms the basis of our analysis was multidisciplinary and included the following Principal Investigators: Ronald Angel, University of Texas at Austin; Linda Burton, Pennsylvania State University; P. Lindsay Chase-Lansdale, Northwestern University; Andrew Cherlin, Johns Hopkins University; Robert Moffitt, Johns Hopkins University; and William Julius Wilson, Harvard University. The following Lead Ethnographers were responsible for collecting the ethnographic data: Laura Lein, University of Texas at Austin; Debra Skinner, University of North Carolina at Chapel Hill; and Constance Willard Williams, Brandeis University. Many other ethnographers, coders, and transcribers assisted in these efforts. A full list of those who participated can be found at the study Web site: http://www.jhu.edu/~welfare/.

A study of this size required a great deal of financial support. Several federal agencies and private foundations contributed generously. Without their support, we could not have carried out the study. We gratefully acknowledge the support of the National Institute of Child Health and Human Development through grants HD36093 and HD25936 and the Office of the Assistant Secretary for Planning and Evaluation, Administration on Developmental Disabilities, Administration for Children and Families, Social Security Administration, National Institute of Mental Health, The Boston Foundation, The Annie E. Casey Foundation, The Edna McConnell Clark Foundation, The Lloyd A. Fry Foundation, Hogg Foundation for Mental Health, The Robert Wood Johnson Foundation, The Joyce Foundation, The Henry J. Kaiser Family Foundation, W. K. Kellogg Foundation,

Kronkosky Charitable Foundation, The John D. and Catherine T. MacArthur Foundation, Charles Stewart Mott Foundation, The David and Lucile Packard Foundation, and Woods Fund of Chicago. We thank Pauline Boss for the insights she gave us during the early stages of developing this book. Finally, we thank the families who graciously participated in the project and gave us access to their lives.

Poor Families in America's Health Care Crisis

The Unrealized Hope of Welfare Reform

Implications for Health Care

Cecilia, a young biracial (African American and Hispanic) mother of two, identified herself as African American. She was introduced to us by another of our San Antonio respondents. We conducted a number of interviews with her over the course of a year and a half, during which her second child, a daughter named Annika, was born. When we met Cecilia, she was living with Annika's father. Her older child, a two-year-old boy named Kevin, was from a previous relationship. Cecilia's own childhood had been chaotic. Her father had thirteen children with various women, but Cecilia only knew two of her siblings and was not particularly close to either of them. One lived in another state and although Cecilia had talked to her on the phone, they had never met in person. Cecilia lived near her mother, but they were not close and Cecilia received little help from her. She described her mother as "remote" and unwilling to provide child care or other assistance to the family.

Cecilia's grandmother also lived nearby, and Cecilia's relationship with her was much warmer than her relationship with her mother. Her grandmother provided what support she could, and Cecilia greatly appreciated the help. When we met Cecilia, she was estranged from Kevin's father and would not allow him to have any contact with the boy. She felt that the father no longer had any right to see his son because he had stopped paying child support. Cecilia seemed resigned to the realities of her life and told us that she had always known that she was going to have to raise her children alone. As she explained,

I made it [the decision to raise the children alone] before my first son was born and I knew I wasn't going to have their dad because he wasn't there when I was pregnant. He wasn't there really. . . . I wanted to show my mom that I can do it as a teen parent. . . . If my partner left me today I'll be alright because I feel like I can do it by myself even though I'm going to still struggle. I can do it myself.

After the birth of her first child, Cecilia quickly discovered that life with an infant was a real struggle. Although Kevin was bright and active, he developed behavioral problems at a very early age and acted up at the day care center where he stayed while Cecilia worked at a fast food restaurant. After he bit several other children, the center staff told Cecilia that she could no longer leave him there. Without child care for Kevin, Cecilia lost her job, and without a job she lost her apartment. She was forced to move back with her mother for a short time before she found another subsidized apartment. Luckily, early in the study, Cecilia was able to move to her own apartment away from her mother and the dangerous neighborhood in which her mother lived. Cecilia expressed great relief at being able to move away from what she described as the ill-behaved children and drug culture of her mother's neighborhood. Her new home was in a pleasantly landscaped compound with electronic access gates.

Cecilia and both children suffered from acute and chronic health problems for which Cecilia struggled to obtain treatment. Cecilia suffered from arthritis, and Kevin experienced frequent asthma attacks. Cecilia's second pregnancy had ended with a protracted labor and a complicated delivery that left her with ongoing medical problems. Like so many of the parents we met, Cecilia had to make difficult choices about who would get health care first, and she devoted much of her time and effort to getting care for her children, while she often delayed attending to her own health care needs.

Cecilia and her children were welfare "cyclers." They applied for Temporary Assistance to Needy Families (TANF) whenever the partner with whom Cecilia was living at the time was laid off or moved out or when Cecilia herself lost whatever job she periodically held. The family cycled off the TANF rolls when Cecilia's partner found a new job and was able to support the family and when her child care arrangements and her own health allowed her to work. The health care problems that resulted from her difficult second pregnancy, including weakness and ongoing infections, made it hard for Cecilia to maintain continuous employment, however, and her unstable employment and cycling in and out of jobs became a continuing reality that affected many aspects of the family's life.

Cecilia could not always understand or comply with the TANF regulations, and the state had sanctioned her for noncompliance several times by reducing or cutting off her benefits completely. She had been sanctioned when she did not report child support from Kevin's father. It was shortly thereafter that the boy's father stopped paying child support, but it was some time before her full TANF benefits were reinstated. At one point, Kevin was dropped from Medicaid when Cecilia missed a well-child checkup for him. On another occasion, the state lowered her food stamp allotment when she could not provide her caseworker with an address for Annika's father. Cecilia told us that on one occasion when she was particularly stressed by her case manager's strident questioning she broke down and cried in his office. The case manager was unmoved and told her that he did not believe that she had no income and threatened to sanction her for not reporting it.

The family depended on Medicaid for whatever care the children received and on a local program that allows family members to receive care for a predetermined minimal payment on their accumulated bill. Because this program did not provide free care but only allowed Cecilia to continue receiving care by making small regular payments on what she owed, there was no real possibility that she could ever pay off her medical debt completely. The more realistic outcome was that the debt would simply grow. Cecilia, like so many other impoverished women who accumulate medical debt, owed hundreds of dollars to the program. Our research with low-income mothers revealed just how difficult it is for them to maintain health care coverage for their families and how much time and attention they must devote to finding and keeping their children's health insurance. It also revealed the nearly impossible task these women, many of whom have serious chronic health problems of their own, face in paying for their health care. Most were unable to do so, and Cecilia's case was again typical. Early in her second pregnancy, the family lost all of its TANF, food stamp, and Medicaid coverage because Cecilia had missed a meeting with her caseworker that was required for recertification. Having

missed the meeting, she had failed to file the required "proof of pregnancy" forms that would have allowed her to retain TANF and the
other benefits for herself and had also failed to provide the information
necessary for her children to continue receiving TANF and Medicaid.

In response, Cecilia resubmitted her documentation and began
working with an advocacy organization to regain her welfare benefits.
The difficult pregnancy made Cecilia's situation urgent, and Cecilia
worked hard to try to regain Medicaid coverage before her second
child's birth. It was unclear from our interviews exactly when she did
regain coverage (Cecilia herself was not certain), but she had the coverage by the time of the delivery, and she and the newborn received
the care they needed. She recounted with some irony how even when
she was visibly in the later stages of pregnancy she had to provide
"documentation" that she was in fact pregnant.

While waiting for her Medicaid coverage to resume, Cecilia delayed
medical care for her son, who needed both dental work and treatment
for a hernia. Luckily, her son's hernia receded without treatment, and
Cecilia was relieved that he did not need expensive medical care that
would have inevitably increased the family's medical debt. The dental
care was simply put off. Unfortunately, a few months after Annika's
birth, Cecilia again lost her son's Medicaid. Evidently, she was not up-
to-date with his inoculations, and his Medicaid coverage was again
canceled. As a result, Cecilia again plunged into a time-consuming
flurry of activity to get her son's coverage reinstated.

During the periods when she was well enough to work, Cecilia held a
series of short-term jobs, none of which offered health insurance. Her
partner never received medical insurance from any of his jobs when
he was living with her. Because nondisabled and nonpregnant adults
who are not receiving TANF do not qualify for Medicaid or any other
public program in Texas except under special circumstances, Cecilia
and her partner had no coverage even when they were employed. Like
other uninsured Americans with low incomes, when they suffered from
health problems they had no options other than charity, going into
debt, or simply forgoing care. For the family, the system of health
care financing for the poor resulted in coverage for the children that
was episodic and difficult to maintain, and coverage for the adults in
the family was nonexistent, except for Cecilia herself when she was
pregnant and eligible for Medicaid.

Toward the end of our time with Cecilia, she was hospitalized twice, once shortly after the birth of her daughter, when an incision opened and became infected, and again a month or two later, when she developed a strep infection and there was concern that the infant might also be infected. Because she did not have health insurance, she again used CareLink, which added to her outstanding medical debt. Cecilia's struggle to provide medical care for herself and her family was a never-ending battle, and after the year and a half we were in contact with the family, we left with no sense of how things could ever improve. When the study ended, Cecilia was continuing to work whenever her health allowed her to do so, but her health remained precarious and maintaining steady employment was difficult. She kept her children enrolled in Medicaid when she could make all of the appointments and could provide the necessary documentation. Often, doing so meant missing work. As with the other families in our study, there was no happy ending to Cecilia's story, nor any sense of closure or resolution. As the children get older and as their eligibility for Medicaid changes, Cecilia's struggle for health care will change as well, but it will never end.

In the following chapters, we tell the stories of other low-income families and their encounters with the health care system and their attempts to obtain and keep medical care coverage. As with Cecilia, most of the stories we heard were confusing in many ways, largely because the lives of the people we worked with were often confusing and chaotic. Unlike fictional accounts, the story plots are not complete and there are often large gaps in the narratives. Although for the most part the mothers we interviewed were remarkably candid about their lives and were forthcoming with information, we could not always be sure when members of the family were employed and when they had health insurance because their lives were simply too complex and confusing to be easily entered into the sort of time and activity matrix that researchers often use (or that a well-crafted novel might portray). Even in directed interviews, the sequence of events and the identification of who did what when was often unclear to us and probably to the mothers themselves.

These families' efforts to obtain and keep continuous health care coverage represent only one of the many domains in which they faced daily struggles. In addition to health care, they had to worry about food, clothing, housing, education, employment, child care, transportation, and much more. Each of these domains presented multiple problems, and they could not be sure from month to month that their needs would be met. It was almost impossible for most to maintain long-term daily routines. Like Cecilia's, the problems they dealt with were rarely fully resolved and they fed upon one another. Our families cycled in and out of jobs and on and off welfare, Medicaid, private insurance, and other programs as numerous other problems impinged on their efforts to maintain their households. We came to realize that even they were frequently unsure as to which members of the family were covered by which programs or whether they were covered at all. Some, for instance, thought their children were covered by Medicaid only to find when they attempted to use medical services that the child was in fact not covered.

The stories we recount represent the best summaries of the lives of these families that we could compile from lengthy narrative interviews. Narrative lacks the neat structure of surveys in which every respondent is asked the same question in the same order and in the same way. It requires interpretation and judgment and in the end provides information that may not be statistically generalizable like that of a survey. On the other hand, narrative provides otherwise unavailable detail on the human experience of dealing with serious adversity in physical and social environments that seem to attack and undermine an impoverished family's every effort to get ahead. These stories are not verbatim transcriptions of what our respondents told us. The narratives were often too long and difficult to follow and much of the verbatim conversation too rambling and unstructured to make sense out of context. The stories we recount summarize, paraphrase, and characterize the lengthy conversations that we had with our respondents. We believe we have stayed true to the content of what our respondents wished to communicate. Of course, we also conducted a survey, and that information tells a similar story, but the narratives provide insight into what lies behind the numbers in a way that only intensive and free-flowing narrative can do.

The Three City Study

The chapters that follow focus on the system of health care coverage for the poor in the United States as it affects families like those in our study. As part of the discussion, we place that system in historical perspective and elaborate the unique situation of the United States among developed nations in not providing health care to all of its citizens as a basic right. As part of the development of our argument in favor of such a universal system, we draw on many data sources. The core of the presentation draws on information from the Three City Study, a large, multidisciplinary examination of the consequences of welfare reform for children and families. The two components of the study that we employ in this book, a survey of 2,400 families in poor neighborhoods in Boston, Chicago, and San Antonio and intensive ethnographic interviews with over 255 families from these same neighborhoods, provide detailed information on health insurance and health care and are described in the context of the larger study.

The larger study consisted of four components: (1) the survey, which was developed by anthropologists, economists, sociologists, and developmental psychologists; (2) an intensive developmental assessment of young children in those same families; (3) an intensive ethnography based on a separate sample of poor families similar in income to those in the survey and who lived in the same neighborhoods from which the survey sample was drawn; and (4) a similar ethnographic study of families that included someone with a significant disability. The logic of this design was to understand the lives of the poor and the potential impact that welfare might have on children from as many salient perspectives as possible. Each discipline and approach provided useful information and insights that informed the interpretation of the data we collected. The study represents a new and powerful approach to understanding complex social phenomena and provides important information that can inform public policy.

The survey consisted of two waves, the first of which was carried out from March to December 1999 in preselected low-income neighborhoods in Boston, Chicago, and San Antonio. As part of the selection criteria, each household contained at least one child younger than four or one child between the ages of ten and fourteen, ages that the developmental psychologists on the team deemed to be of particular developmental importance. Most households, of course, included other children as well. Forty percent of the survey families were receiving cash assistance at the time of the initial interview and, as we will see, very few had private or nongovernmental health insurance. We collected in the survey extensive information on income, education, earnings, employment, health, private health care coverage, Medicaid, welfare use, social program participation, and much more for each household. The second survey was conducted between September 2000 and May 2001 and collected information concerning changes in such factors as household structure, insurance coverage, and health care since the first interview. A third wave is in the field as this book goes to press. In what follows, we use information from the first and second waves of the survey to frame and generalize the discoveries from the ethnographic component.

The ethnography included a series of open-ended interviews and observations in the homes of mothers and their children in the same neighborhoods in which the survey was conducted, although the ethnographic families were not among those surveyed. The families that participated in the ethnography had household incomes of no more than 200 percent of the federal poverty line (FPL). The ethnographic sample design called for interviewers to recruit sixty families in each city from among each of three racial and ethnic groups: African Americans, Hispanics, and non-Hispanic whites. A smaller group of families that included someone with a serious disability was also selected. The study plan called for each interviewer to work with about six or seven families, visiting each family once a month for discussions of a variety of issues, including child-rearing practices and family rituals, the education and work histories of household members, and health and medical care coverage. Data were collected over a three-year period from 1999 to 2002. Interviews and observations were transcribed and coded and then entered into a qualitative database.

The ethnographic families were contacted between June 1999 and December 2000. About 40 percent of the families researched were Hispanic, 40 percent African American, and 20 percent non-Hispanic white, and roughly equal numbers came from the three study cities. To the extent possible, ethnographers met with each family an average of once or twice a month for between twelve and eighteen months and then again approximately six months and twelve months later. Although most meetings occurred in respondents' homes, the ethnographers also accompanied members of the families to the grocery store, family celebrations, welfare offices, and on a number of other family errands and activities. Topics addressed during these ethnographic visits with families included health and health care access, experiences with social welfare agencies, education and training, work experiences and plans, family budgets and economic strategies, parenting and child development, and support networks, among other issues. The work with families was accompanied by extensive neighborhood ethnographies in which ethnographers collected information on neighborhood resources (Burton et al. 2001; Winston et al. 1999).

The location and recruitment of families, the interview process, and the efforts to retain the families' involvement throughout the project illustrate many of the difficulties of intensive research with families in poverty as well as the nature of their life circumstances. We recruited families in neighborhoods that were home to impoverished families, and the families themselves had household incomes below 200 percent of FPL. In earlier work, we learned that families are most likely to participate fully in research of this nature if they are introduced to the project and the researchers by a trusted intermediary (Edin and Lein 1997). For that reason, the interviewers recruited families through public housing offices, day care centers, clinics, educational programs, and other contacts in the community.

We did not, however, recruit among the poorest of the poor. Interviewers did not seek out families in homeless shelters, in halfway houses, at centers that provided services for victims of domestic violence, or in situations where the children had been removed by the authorities. The mothers who participated in the study were women who were likely to have at least temporarily stable addresses, ties to at least one community organization, and a family consisting of at least the mother and a child. Many of the families in the study were struggling, but they were not the truly down-and-out. On the other hand, because we were recruiting families in low-income neighborhoods, neither did the study include families who were financially successful enough to move out. However, other studies of low-income families, particularly those drawing on large administrative databases, find that very few families actually move out of poverty in the years after they leave the welfare rolls (Isaacs and Lyon 2000; Schexnayder et al. 2002). In many ways, the families we studied resemble the more narrowly defined group of welfare leavers described in these studies in that they usually had some experience with one or another welfare program, they lived in a poor neighborhood, and their work experience was characterized by unstable jobs and low wages.

We can usefully describe our sample of families as a "middle cut" of low-wage and unemployed families. The families we describe were certainly struggling. Most were barely making ends meet, they were cycling between jobs and unemployment, and most were often behind in paying their bills. As we shall see, they often experienced lapses in health insurance, they had problems with housing, and they had difficulty paying for food, utilities, and transportation. However, in most cases, mothers and children were still together, and many found periods of stability that punctuated the periods of crisis and ongoing chaos that permeated much of their lives.

Even this middle-cut group of families experienced pressures, tensions, and discontinuities that took them out of the research process for a time, often leaving us with an incomplete record of their experiences. As we noted earlier, our original plan called for interviewing families on at least a monthly basis for eighteen months. However, only a minority of the families were available on a regular basis over the entire eighteen-month period. Thus, there are often blanks in our record of the families' life experiences. Families that experienced a sudden eviction (a more common event in Texas than in the other states because of the lack of tenant protection regulations), a sudden critical medical crisis, or any of a number of other setbacks were often difficult to find and unavailable for participation in the research project for a period of time. However, it was important to the nature of this research to keep these families in our sample. If we had excluded all families for whom there were discontinuities and missing data, our conclusions would have been based on an atypically stable group of poor families.

We also found that family life was sufficiently complicated that, on occasion, families did not know the answers to questions that, at least during the planning phase of the project, had seemed straightforward. These included such questions as whether the respondent was employed. The women in our study, like those in other studies of marginal workers, experienced frequent periods of unemployment and job hunting. For days, or even weeks, they might have been under the impression that they had their next job lined up. In such situations, they may well have told the interviewer that they were employed, even though they had not yet worked or received their first paycheck. Health insurance was also confusing. The complexity of the application and recertification process for Medicaid often led to misinformation concerning a family's status. We found, for example, that a mother might think that her child had Medicaid coverage because she had filled out the application and been told that she was eligible. However, when the child needed medical care, some mothers found out at the provider's office that the child's coverage had not been approved. Upon returning to the Medicaid office, many mothers found that their file was incomplete and missing a critical piece of documentation or that the application had simply not been processed yet.

Another complicated set of issues related to the amount of the family's welfare benefit. The amount of the welfare payment varied from month to month, often for unpredictable reasons. Unforeseen changes in family circumstances, a parent's inability to meet all the welfare requirements, and delays and errors at the welfare office, among other complications and problems, all contributed to variations in welfare payments. Mothers found it difficult to predict their welfare payments or to explain past payments. As a result of all of this complexity, almost every family's narrative includes holes. As we describe families, we will indicate where information is missing.

Because we were intimately involved in the San Antonio component of the ethnography, we draw heavily from those interviews, although we use survey and ethnographic data from the other sites as well. Our focus on San Antonio is also motivated by the fact that Texas has the highest number of uninsured children and adults in the nation and the fact that it serves as an example of the dilemma that arises from the combination of an employment-based health insurance system, a shift in employment toward service-sector jobs that do not provide benefits, and the inability or unwillingness of legislatures to raise taxes.

Although many of the differences among families we document can be traced to different state and local policies, in the ethnography some of the differences among cities probably reflect variations in the way families were recruited. In San Antonio, most families were recruited through public housing programs and multiservice community organizations. In Chicago, families were more likely to be recruited through Head Start programs. In Boston, they were more likely to be recruited through child care centers. In all cases, these families were in contact with public agencies, and in the case of Chicago they were connected with a service, Head Start, which serves only a minority of eligible families. It is therefore clear that these families were all savvy enough and energetic enough to connect with service agencies. Various state characteristics also influenced the research process itself. San Antonio families presented the greatest challenges to the research project because of their high rate of residential mobility. The San Antonio families experienced more evictions and other changes in their housing situations than did families in the two other cities. This was related, at least in part, to the speed with which landlords can evict tenants in Texas. In Massachusetts, and to some extent in Illinois, tenants enjoy greater protection from eviction.

Although the families we studied were not those that were most down-and-out, and although they were attached to helping agencies, they all experienced the unpredictable instabilities of life at the economic margin. Families in Boston were doing marginally better than families in Illinois or Texas. Again, this to some extent reflects the fact that they were recruited through child care centers, they lived in a state with high welfare benefits, and that there were a variety of local health services available to them. As the data we present later reveal, parents in families that used child care centers were more likely to be engaged in somewhat stable employment. In the end, however, the variations among the three cities were of relatively small scale compared with the major impacts of poverty and instability.

Understanding Instability: The Need for Qualitative Research

Although our core focus consists of the nature and consequences of the fragmented and incomplete health care financing system upon which low-income families depend, very early in the study we realized that problems related to health pervaded the lives of the families we studied as well as the narratives they provided. It was immediately obvious that the means-tested nature of the health care and other support systems that they relied upon, and the fact that the requirements of those organizations were often seriously incompatible with work and the ability to establish family routines, meant that these families lived with constant uncertainty and instability. They could take very little for granted from month to month or even week to week. Their incomes varied widely, they remained on waiting lists for subsidized housing for years while they lived in demoralizing conditions, their access to adequate nutrition was often tenuous, and their health care coverage was uncertain. Such instability can undermine the most sincere efforts to achieve self-sufficiency of even the most functional family and the most psychologically resilient parents. The theme of instability is therefore necessarily central to our story, and in order to illustrate how instability pervades the lives of low-income families, we must show how instability in health care is related to and exacerbates instability in all other areas of the lives of low-income families. Our task is to make some sense of the instability of the lives we recount and to relate that instability to the institutional and social structures that seriously limit the opportunities for social advancement of families that find themselves at the economic margin.

Alice O'Connor (O'Connor 2001) points out that today researchers who study poverty are in much the same situation as their progressive-era predecessors of over a century earlier. They face the challenge of shifting the focus of research away from a concern with the characteristics and behaviors of poor individuals and families and onto the nature of the economic system that seems to make poverty inevitable. As O'Connor and others point out, since the 1960s the study of poverty has become extremely sophisticated. Methodological innovations based on major data-collection efforts, including income maintenance experiments, large-scale social surveys, and advanced statistical modeling techniques have provided very useful insights that have put simplistic explanations of the causes of poverty to rest. A long tradition of quantitative work focuses on issues related to employment, income, program participation, and other characteristics of individuals and families that move on or off the cash assistance rolls (Braumer and Loprest 1999; Isaacs and Lyon 2000; Moffitt 1992; Moffitt and Winder 2003a; Moffitt and Winder 2003b). It is clear by now that the rise in single motherhood, the decay of our inner cities, and poverty are part of a complex set of social changes that are global in nature. Only the most intransigent ideologue would still contend that welfare is the sole and direct cause of single motherhood or the decline of the family.

For the most part, research on poverty has been quantitative, with the occasional addition of a qualitative component, and most of the policy debate has been informed by quantitative studies. The power of quantification and the scientific legitimacy that it conveys in discussions of social issues makes it the dominant methodology in American social science. Yet even sophisticated quantitative researchers are well aware of the limitations of self-reported information and of the shortcomings of administrative data. Explanations of poverty, single motherhood, and social disorder usually focus on norms and complex social processes whose impact can only be imprecisely understood with survey data. Processes that are by their very nature highly contextual can only be understood in context (Berick 1995; Hays 2003; Loury 2001; Rank 1994). Even economists recognize the importance of noneconomic factors on entry into and exit from welfare, including the impact of state administrative differences and implementation barriers (Bell 2001; Blank 2002; Moffitt 2003a). Yet for the most part the noneconomic aspects of poverty receive little policy attention.

Welfare reform was motivated in large part by the widespread perception that the old approach was a failure and was doing more harm than good both to individuals and society (Heclo 2001; Mead 2001; Sawhill 1995). Part of the concern focused on the behavior of the poor, including their fertility behavior, an aspect of life that is no doubt influenced by income but is also driven by much more that the economic focus does not address. In order to understand these complex contextualized social processes, one must employ approaches other than survey research. Poor families live in cultural and social environments in which multiple factors influence their capacity for instrumental action. If one has little control over important aspects of one's life, one must devote a great deal of time and energy to obtaining the basic necessities of daily living. One can take very little for granted because problems are not solved for the long term but only for the short run. Often individuals in such situations engage in actions that might seem irrational or self-destructive to an outside observer. For instance, difficulties in obtaining insurance and paying for care often lead to the neglect of one's health, which can undermine employment and family stability.

An ethnographic perspective illuminates the multiple and complex causes and consequences of the *instability* of employment and income in the lives of the poor with the sort of comprehensive detail that quantitative survey-based research cannot approximate. Certainly instability in employment manifests itself as a low number of hours worked per week or moving through multiple jobs during a relatively short period. Yet a variety of underlying processes can give rise to similar statistical profiles. Ethnography allows us to closely examine family life and to understand the causes of instability in work, and it reveals how instability in employment is related to instability in other areas of family life. Ethnography reveals how family, work, and health problems evolve in an iterative process that feeds back upon itself, often resulting in a cascade of negative outcomes. Our ethnographic interviews allowed us to gain insights as to why poor families manage to gain only very limited control over many aspects of family life, including their access to health insurance and regular health care.

Of course, it is certainly not the case that qualitative research on poverty has been completely ignored. Several excellent studies clearly demonstrate the depth of understanding of the everyday life of the poor that only intensive participation can reveal (Angel and Lein forthcoming; Berick 1995; Burton, Lein, and Kolak 2005; Edin and Kefalas 2005; Edin and Lein 1997; Garey 1999; Hays 2003; Henly and Lyons 2000; Kingfisher 1996; Lein et al. 2005; Newman 1999; Newman 2001; Rank 1994; Stack 1997). Increasingly, researchers and policy analysts are becoming aware of the necessity of combining quantitative and qualitative methodologies and of paying more attention to those outside of the academic world who have knowledge of the bureaucracies that the poor must negotiate (Loury 2001; O'Connor 2001). Quantitative studies provide information on the patterning of social phenomena; qualitative studies provide deeper insights into the forces that give rise to those patterns and the subjective reality that lies behind them.

The Elusiveness of Daily Routines

Cecilia's situation was typical of that of the families that we got to know while carrying out our research. For families at the economic margin, the availability of medical care coverage, as well as the availability of other necessities of life, depends on whether a mother or her partner are employed and the kinds of jobs they hold. As we quickly found out, steady employment is a major challenge for poor families, and the ability to find and keep a job depends on many other factors, including the ability to find child care during the hours that parents are required to work, the unexpected illness of a family member that can cause a parent to lose her job, the time demands required by the process of applying for or recertifying one's eligibility for TANF, Medicaid, food stamps, or other programs, the availability of transportation, and much more.

For the families we studied, few areas of life were predictable or the same from week to week, and the accumulated unpredictability made it difficult for them to establish routines. None of our families had a breadwinner who had a long-term, stable job with a consistent and predictable schedule and a basic package of benefits. Of course, such families were unlikely to have ended up in our sample. The lives of most of our families embodied the contradictions of life at the economic margin and on a daily basis revealed the pitfalls of poorly informed expectations for welfare reform. For most of our families, unemployment or episodic employment was the norm and self-sufficiency an elusive goal that formal welfare policy itself, of which health care policy is a good example, made even more unattainable.

The basic objective of welfare reform, even putting aside unrealistic expectations of economic self-sufficiency, was to encourage, or rather force, parents who receive cash assistance to assume greater responsibility for their own economic well-being and that of their children. Unless they are disabled or retired, most American adults work and support their families. For most of us, the hours we spend at work take up a major part of our lives. One's occupation, along with one's age, forms an integral part of one's identity and self-concept and serves as the foundation of our social definition of responsible citizenship. Welfare reform made that expectation explicit for the recipients of publicly funded cash assistance, and the legislation had broad support (Mead 2001; Teles 1996). The enabling legislation was ultimately signed into law by Democratic president Bill Clinton, the leader of the party traditionally viewed as supporting welfare, and it was impossible to deny that the time for a major change in American welfare policy had arrived (Heclo 2001; Mead 2001; O'Connor 2001). The welfare recipients who participated in the focus groups that were part of the planning for this study shared in the expectation that adults should support themselves, and they expressed a sincere desire to do so themselves (Burton et al. 1988).

Yet even as the poor affirm the core American values of work and self-sufficiency, they face immense challenges in conforming to those values. Decades of research on poverty also make it clear that the challenges they face are not the result of welfare reform. In the end, the radical changes that were part of the new legislation may make little long-term difference. The challenges that poor families face existed before welfare reform was conceived of, and they remain even after it supposedly ended welfare as we knew it. The barriers to social mobility that the poor encounter are part of the very structure of the worlds of work and family life in which they live and from which they find it difficult to escape. Our ethnographic data provide insights into those barriers that challenge simplistic notions of personal irresponsibility.

Our data show that unemployed and low-income parents face a daunting number of barriers in their efforts to maintain the routines of work and family life that characterize the middle class in America. Cecilia did her best to combine her responsibilities to her young children with paid employment. Some critics might fault her efforts or deny that she had any real desire to get ahead, but as we got to know her and her children and the other families in the study, we learned that her situation was at times chaotic in ways over which she had little real control. She and her family cycled on and off welfare as work and partners came and went, and while we were in contact with her she never managed to settle into a long-term sustainable routine of work and family life. For families like Cecilia's, the basic requirements for sustainable routines, including regular employment, dependable transportation, reliable and affordable child care, and good health care were unattainable over the long run. At the same time that Cecilia had to juggle work and her other family responsibilities, her own and her children's health problems, and the difficulties in getting medical insurance and treatment for them, were an ever-present barrier to her ability to gain control over her life. The instability that plagued much of the rest of her life played itself out in continuing lapses in health insurance for one or another member of her family.

Family Life without Health Care Coverage

The lack of consistent health care coverage and the consequent ongoing scramble to maintain it and to get medical care was a major source of instability and uncertainty in the lives of the families we studied. The fundamental problem of coverage for the working poor lies in the very nature of the tax-subsidized, employer-based health insurance system unique to the United States (Enthoven 1978; Reinhardt 1998). Few, if any, of our families had breadwinners with stable jobs that offered health insurance at a price the family could afford. Most workers in the families we met were not offered health insurance plans at all. For many of our families, the poor health of one or more members began a downward spiral that increased the family's instability, undermined their income-generating strategies, and sometimes drove them further into poverty. Parents with low-wage service-sector jobs very often lose those jobs when they become ill, and given the nearly complete absence of public health coverage for adults, they often go without care themselves even when they manage to get it for their children. Our interviews revealed that, even for families that escape the downward spiral, the lack of health care coverage and its consequences have serious ramifications for family indebtedness, health status, and future employment opportunities.

A large body of research makes it clear that insurance matters and that the poor face a double jeopardy in that they are both at higher risk of illness and are less likely to receive adequate care than the middle class. The literature provides extensive evidence that poverty has significant negative consequences for all aspects of physical and emotional health (Institute of Medicine 2002a; Link and Phelan 2002; Phillips 2003). Low-income families suffer more illness and more serious types of illness than do families that are better-off (Williams and Collins 1995). Entire neighborhoods in the socially and economically impoverished areas of our large cities have poorer overall health profiles than better-off neighborhoods (Winkleby and Cubbins 2003). Certain groups in our study were at particularly high risk of the illnesses associated with poverty. For instance, the prevalence of diabetes continues to rise dramatically for all Americans, but it is particularly high among Mexican Americans, who make up the largest Hispanic group in our study (Bastida, Cuéllar, and Villas, 2001; Carter, Pugh, and Monterrosa 1996; Stern et al. 1992; Vinicor 1994).

At the same time that the poor suffer from more frequent and more serious acute and chronic illnesses, their lack of health care coverage, or their incomplete coverage, is a clear health risk. There is ample evidence showing that health insurance is associated with better health (Institute of Medicine 2001). The children in our study families suffered from all of the health conditions that are increasingly prevalent among low-income children, including asthma, ear infections, allergies, bronchitis, and obesity. The adults suffered from what are rapidly becoming the chronic conditions of the poor, including obesity, hypertension, and diabetes. Although charity coverage is sometimes available, and even though the poor often receive care in emergency rooms, that care is hardly the continuous and complete care that defines the best medicine. Low-income individuals without health insurance see physicians far less often, are less likely to have a regular source of care, and are more likely to do without care than individuals with insurance (Aday, Fleming, and Andersen 1984; Ayanian et al. 1993; Ayanian et al. 2000; Baker, Shapiro, and Schur 2000; Freeman et al. 1990; Haley and Zuckerman 2000; Institute of Medicine 2001; Zweifel and Manning 2000). Individuals without insurance are more likely to die of cancer and other serious diseases because of late diagnoses and inadequate care (Ayanian et al. 1993; Pepper Commission 1990; Roetzheim et al. 2000).

The uninsured not only suffer from poorer health than the insured but also incur greater costs for the services they use because they are subject to a 100 percent co-payment because they must pay the full cost of whatever care they receive. The uninsured also often pay more for medical care than those with group insurance because they do not benefit from the discounts negotiated by employers and large insurers (Wielawski 2000). Medicaid clearly makes up for some of these deficits for families who qualify. Children enrolled in Medicaid are more likely to receive preventive and acute health care than those who are not enrolled, and their families incur fewer out-of-pocket expenses (Davidoff, Garrett, and Schirmer 2000; Kasper, Giovannini, and Hoffman 2000; Ku and Blaney 2000). Emergency rooms and local and state programs also assume part of the bill. However, the inability to maintain Medicaid or other coverage, which our study reveals to be a major problem for unemployed or low-wage families, has potentially serious negative consequences for family health, employment, income, and stability.

What the research shows is that the combination of impoverishment and the bureaucratic complications experienced by many poor families in disorganized urban neighborhoods creates conditions that increase the risk of illness and results in the delay of treatment. The combination of these increased health risks and irregular and inadequate health care means that the families that live in these situations must cope with more health problems for longer periods than those with more resources who live in more affluent social and physical environments.

The Policy Context of Family Health Care Coverage

Although this book was motivated by a desire to assess the impact of welfare reform on health care coverage for low-income families, in the end we were inevitably forced to deal with the entire complexity of the lives of the families we studied and the forces that undermined their attempts to establish routines and build longer-term economic security. Our interviews made it clear that health and health care financing problems were integrally related to a complex set of other difficulties, but the core problem as it related to health care coverage and the basic focus of the book can be stated quite simply: In the United States, the richest nation in the world and with the most technically advanced medical care system in existence, low-income families are unable to obtain and keep continuous health care coverage for all members of their households. Unemployed and working poor families face periods, sometimes quite long, during which some of their children, and very often one or more adults, have no health care coverage. The well-documented connection between health care coverage, health care use, and health outcomes that we mentioned earlier means that unequal access to health care coverage contributes directly to inequalities in health and well-being (Institute of Medicine 2001; Institute of Medicine 2002a). These inequalities are not simply unfair; they pose serious practical problems for our nation's future economic and social stability.

Although it is clear that welfare reform, at least initially, significantly reduced Medicaid participation by poor families, the incomplete and discontinuous nature of health insurance coverage for low-income families has its roots far deeper in poverty, the employment-based nature of the health insurance system of the United States, and, ultimately, in the often contradictory combination of labor force, welfare, and health care policies themselves. Furthermore, although welfare reform, Medicaid, and the new State Children's Health Insurance Program (SCHIP) were implemented differently in each state, all state health care financing systems are based on similar basic assumptions and common federal guidelines. Any discussion of health care for the poor brings one face-to-face with the health care consequences of our reliance on a means-tested health care insurance approach for the poor rather than a system of universal coverage. It also forces one to question the limits of incremental and piecemeal reforms. Our review of the literature on the health care difficulties of the poor and near-poor, in addition to our own interviews, made it clear that the crisis of health care coverage is growing and that a growing fraction of the working poor and even members of the middle class find it difficult to obtain and afford adequate and continuous family coverage. What we illustrate with detailed survey and ethnographic data is that for the working poor the nature of work and the nature of health care contribute in an interactive manner to economic instability and to frequent cycling in and out of poverty.

Our ethnographic data made it clear that this cycling resulted from the interconnectedness of sources of family instability. To one degree or another, uncertainty and instability were inevitable aspects of life for all of the families in our sample. As we illustrate in the subsequent chapters, illness struck unexpectedly, breadwinners lost their jobs from one day to the next, and circumstances beyond the family's control often meant disaster. Families' lack of economic reserves or dependable support meant that small problems frequently escalated into serious crises. Yet despite serious economic vulnerabilities and frequent crises, some families seemed to function well. They possessed certain family and social resources that helped them cope, or they may simply have been lucky and healthy. If setbacks were rare or if they occurred in isolation from one another, a family was sometimes able to cope, especially if they had some savings and other material or social resources. If crises occurred together or in rapid succession, or if instability pervaded family life, problems often cascaded and undermined all options for family stability and upward mobility.

In the following chapters, we focus on instability in health insurance coverage among poor families and illustrate the complex associations between the precariousness of health coverage and the instability of employment experienced by low-wage families. We also illustrate the fact that minority-group status, defined in terms of race and ethnicity, interacts with other structural factors related to work and the availability of health benefits to place African Americans and Hispanics at particularly high risk of lacking health coverage (De la Torre 1996; Doty 2003). We show, however, that the most serious barriers to

adequate coverage arise from the interaction of formal welfare policy
and the employment options available to the working poor that create
an environment characterized by instability and unpredictability that
undermines even heroic efforts at family stability, let alone economic
mobility.

Jobs with No Stability and No Health Insurance

Workers with low educational levels and few job skills find themselves
confined to the growing service sector, in which jobs are often characterized by instability in hours, wages, and job tenure and in which wages
can fluctuate unpredictably. These workers, who are disproportionately African American and Latino, often experience frequent periods
of underemployment and unemployment. Few receive employer-
sponsored health insurance as a benefit, and even if they do, the premiums and co-payment requirements place family coverage out of reach of
most low-wage workers. Even under the constraints of welfare reform,
many families continue to cycle on and off welfare and, partly as a consequence, to cycle on and off Medicaid. Because of different eligibility
criteria for younger and older children, some family members cycle at
different rates and times than others. This situation clearly undermines
the possibility for stability or the ability to plan.

The jobs that low-wage workers are able to find deviate considerably from the model of regular nine-to-five jobs that most of us consider
stable employment. Yet the extent and nature of the fundamental instability of low-wage work and its impact on family life is often hidden
behind the almost exclusive focus on income and labor supply that is
typical of most of the large-scale survey-based statistical evaluations
that dominate welfare and labor force policy analysis (Acs, Loprest,
and Roberts 2001; Blank and Schmidt 2001; Heclo 2001; Loprest 2002;
Loprest 2003b; Moffitt 2003a; Moffitt 2003b; O'Connor 2001). Wages
and hours worked are clearly important aspects of jobs, but anyone
who has worked knows that a job brings much more into one's life
than money and requires much more than time. Work, or the lack of
it, has a major impact on one's life in many noneconomic ways. However, because income is clearly a central motivation for working and is
indisputably an important determinant of one's quality of life, a focus
on money and hours worked makes sense.

However, through our ethnographic interviews, we came to realize that the instability of work in and of itself has negative consequences above and beyond those related to hours and wages. The parents we interviewed structured, or were unable to structure, their work lives in an environment in which jobs were often hard to get and easy to lose. They had little control over how and when they would work because an employer might demand irregular hours or rotating shifts. Schedules and the money they earned changed by the week, or even by the day. Such jobs undermine a family's ability to maintain routines and regularity, including regularity of health insurance and health care, and the instability of any one job makes it difficult to combine multiple jobs in order to increase family income. Among our respondents, child care needs, sleep times, meal times, and transportation patterns all varied with the demands of unpredictable jobs. Such pressured and irregular lives provided little time and few opportunities for adults to enhance their human capital and get training, education, and experience with new skills in ways that might help the family to move out of poverty on a permanent basis. Although the prevalence of these problems may have increased with the onset of welfare reform, they have their origins in policies and institutional structures, including those revolving around health care and health insurance, that precede the reforms of the 1990s.

The Racial and Ethnic Factor

Since the introduction of Social Security in the 1930s and Medicare in the 1960s, poverty and the lack of health care coverage have shifted from problems that once plagued the elderly to major problems for young working poor families with children (Myles 1989; Quadagno 1988a; U.S. Bureau of the Census 1998). Today poverty is concentrated among families with young children, and an increasing number of these families are headed by a single female (U.S. Bureau of the Census 2003a). The poor are also disproportionately African American and Hispanic. Figure 1.1 shows that in 2003 33 percent of African American children and 29 percent of Hispanic children lived in families with incomes below the official poverty cutoff. These proportions were three times those of non-Hispanic white children, 10 percent of whom lived in families with incomes below the poverty level. Of course, given

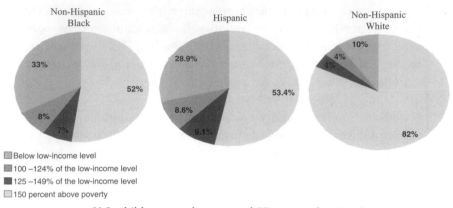

Non-Hispanic Black

Hispanic

Non-Hispanic White

☐ Below low-income level
■ 100 –124% of the low-income level
■ 125 –149% of the low-income level
☐ 150 percent above poverty

FIGURE 1.1. U.S. child poverty by race and Hispanic ethnicity. Source: 2003 Current Population Survey (March), U.S. Bureau of the Census.

the overwhelming size of the non-Hispanic population, the majority of the poor are non-Hispanic whites. Nonetheless, the fact that a disproportionate fraction of the poor are African American and Hispanic has had important implications for the evolution of U.S. welfare policy (Quadagno 1988a; Quadagno 1988b; Quadagno 1994; Weir, Orloff, and Skocpol 1988).

There can be little doubt that welfare policy and our public attitudes toward the poor have been influenced by our history of racial conflict and discrimination (Bonilla-Silva 2003; Gilens 1999; Lieberman 1998; Quadagno 1994; Weir, Orloff, and Skocpol 1988). Media coverage of the most negative and unappealing aspects of welfare and poverty have focused disproportionately on minority Americans and public support for antipoverty programs has been declining since they became associated with African American and inner-city poverty (Gilens 1999; Heclo 1995; Heclo 2001). The issue of race has always been divisive, and even many liberals wish that the topic could be laid to rest (Bonilla-Silva 2003; Schlesinger 1992). Clearly, many of the problems of African Americans and Hispanics result from education, employment, and language problems that leave them outside the economic mainstream (Wilson 1978; Wilson 1987). Yet their unique vulnerabilities reflect the continuing structural disadvantages certain groups face, related in part to subtle forms of institutionalized racism rather than overt bigotry (Bonilla-Silva 2003). It is impossible to discuss the situation of poor families without dealing with the issue of race and ethnicity. Our survey sample, like our ethnographic sample, was primarily African American and Hispanic, a fact that reflects our sample design but even more so the fact that poor urban neighborhoods are disproportionately minority.

The new age-based shift in the burden of poverty from the elderly to families with children takes on a distinctly racial and ethnic dimension because a disproportionate number of poor families are African American and Hispanic. As we document in the following chapters, race and ethnicity, although often left out of the discussion, pervade one's experiences, and they affect where families live and work and, consequently, whether they have health insurance and if and where they get health care. Today the vast majority of poor children qualify for Medicaid or SCHIP, yet many do not enroll even though they qualify (Dubay, Haley, and Kenney 2002; Guyer 2000; Perry et al. 2000). This fact reflects many complex factors related to poverty and the bureaucratic complexity involved in the application and recertification procedures. Many of these factors are related to the social and political barriers associated with being African American or Hispanic. Discussing race and ethnicity as if they were separate from and independent of socioeconomic and other barriers to economic success and continuous health care misrepresents reality. In the United States today, minority-group status, especially for African Americans and certain Hispanics, places one at high risk of poverty and its negative consequences, including a lack of health insurance and difficulty accessing health care.

We Are Mexicans

To be "Mexican" in San Antonio is to live in a city replete with the symbols of one's culture of origin. Non-Hispanics have adopted Mexican dress and food and the beauty and ease with which they fit the geography and culture of the Southwest. To grow up a Mexican in San Antonio or any other American city, however, means that even as one participates in the economic life of the larger society, one remains conscious of one's difference. This fact is rarely articulated in everyday interactions or even in our ethnographic interviews. Ethnicity seems too basic an aspect of identity to require, or even lend itself to, verbal expression. Overt ethnic consciousness largely remains confined to the realm of political discourse, often of a confrontational nature. Yet the events of our families' daily lives were conditioned to one degree or another by the fact that they were "Mexican" and therefore, depending on their social class, education, skin color, dress, and more, different from the "Anglo," a term that refers to the large heterogeneous group of non-Mexicans whose defining characteristic is that they are the group with the greatest economic and political power.

In the Southwest, the Mexican and Anglo cultures have over the years evolved a degree of mutually beneficial rapprochement such that intermarriage between members of these groups presents fewer serious social difficulties than an interracial marriage. Even in the absence of an articulated consciousness of their Mexican ethnicity, however, for those with few resources, the fact of belonging to this specific group pervades everything they do. In Chicago, in which the large Mexican arrival is much more recent, the cultural distance is probably even greater. For our families with little money or social standing, it was difficult not to be conscious of the differences between themselves and others in social interactions, even when those differences went unspoken. As we learned from our interviews, in interactions with authorities and institutions, the families we spoke with could not help but be conscious of the fact that most of the clients with whom they shared the waiting room were Mexican or black. The fact that the caseworker might be a minority-group member as well did not alter this reality, nor did it alter their position in relation to the authority he or she represented. The system as a whole is defined by the Anglo, to whom they must continuously appeal for the necessities of life, often sacrificing elements of their basic dignity in the process. This degradation is a theme to which they return frequently in our discussions.

The Need for a New Discourse on Poverty and Health Care

Our fundamental argument is that academic researchers and public policymakers have not focused sufficiently on the impact of instability and the lack of routines on all aspects of poor families' lives or on the role of poor health and the lack of health care coverage in exacerbating that instability. Ultimately, we see no solution to this major social problem and personal tragedy other than a fully funded, federally mandated, universal system of basic health care coverage. As we argue in Chapter 8, piecemeal and partial reforms may be an inevitable first step, but a continuation of the current system that focuses on work solutions and coercive welfare policies will never address the health care coverage problems of the poor.

The nation's experience with welfare since the 1960s has shown that the problems of poverty cannot be overcome by simple policies and programs, and it is unlikely that in the future policies based on coercion will be any more effective. The poor do not have to be forced to work; they almost uniformly express the desire to work and demonstrate the sincerity of that desire on a daily basis by taking low-paying jobs with little autonomy or benefits. Like members of the middle class, the working poor need jobs that provide a living wage and that provide them access to basic health care and other human services that would allow them to maintain their basic dignity.

One of the motivations for requiring the recipients of cash assistance to work was the belief that working parents are better role models for their children. Hardly anyone would argue that a family in which one or both parents work at a good job is better off in every regard than a family that must rely on charity. But work that by its very nature undermines self-confidence and undermines family stability and routines may well undermine the goal of strengthening families. Although our focus is primarily on health insurance, the issues of poverty, like the issue of race, simply cannot be ignored. Our study led us to conclude that, to a large extent, the failure of the old AFDC cash assistance system, and the potential failure of the reformed system, results from the failure of public policy to deal adequately with the nonwage elements of work and the noneconomic aspects of poverty and family life. Among the most important of those is health and inadequate health care coverage.

Someone's Care Must Be Sacrificed

The incomplete system of coverage that we observed required that families engage in a form of medical care triage on their own. Although mothers were usually successful in enrolling their children in Medicaid, albeit often with frequent lapses, they were likely to neglect their own health and often did not get the medical care they needed because they used their limited resources of time and money for other purposes. Unless a woman is pregnant or very ill, she does not independently qualify for health care under any program. Many of the women we interviewed described a lack of routine and ongoing health care in combination with heavy family and work responsibilities that clearly undermined their physical and mental health. A lack of control over one's own health can result in neglect and the absence of preventive care. Such neglect undermines health and adds a further source of uncertainty to life. If a single mother becomes too ill to work or misses too much work, she may well lose her major source of income.

Most of the mothers we talked to had periods when they neglected their own physical and mental health needs at least to some degree in order to provide for the needs of their children and other family members. When mothers lacked insurance, seeking care for themselves simply involved too many administrative hurdles and complications, as well as financial burdens, and consequently they often went without needed care. Even though many of the mothers received some support for medical expenses and some were at least partially covered on plans owned by their spouses, partners, or the fathers of their children, most told us of times when they tended to simply ignore symptoms and postpone regular checkups. They also often delayed the treatment of serious illnesses until the symptoms began to interfere with their ability to take care of their children and other family members. For these women, health care was often sought only as part of a medical crisis.

One of the most poignant findings of our study was the magnitude of the debt that poor families incurred as the result of illness (Edin and Lein 1997). Because of their poverty and the conditions in which they live and work, the poor are at elevated risk of illness, yet they are also at elevated risk of lacking family health care coverage. This health care double jeopardy means that the more frequent illnesses and the gaps in health insurance that poor families experience almost assure that they will go into debt for needed health care at some time in their lives. Given the high cost of medical care and the rapidity with which medical debts build up during an emergency, a family can very quickly find itself deeply in debt. With limited earnings and many competing demands, the likelihood that such debt will ever be paid off is small. Again, what this means is that illness and the lack of health care coverage for both the mothers and their children made up a large part of the complex of family financial uncertainty, and health problems, health insurance problems, and indebtedness all interacted with work problems to increase many families' lack of control over their life situations. Without reliable health insurance, even a middle-class family is extremely vulnerable to disaster in the event of serious medical problems. For the poor, routine medical problems can be disastrous. Health insurance became an important employment benefit for the middle class after World War II as medical progress and medical care costs introduced economic risks that became too great for even people with substantial savings to bear (Starr 1982). The combination of the inability of parents in poor families to get routine health care and treatment for illnesses when they arise and relentless responsibilities for family members often results in a vicious cycle of more serious illness and growing medical debt. Such a situation can easily spiral out of control. It is hard to see how any of the health care financing reforms, such as medical savings accounts, that have been proposed in recent years could address the health care needs of these families. Market mechanisms are not likely to provide all of the health care that low-wage workers need at a price they can even begin to afford. As medical inflation outstrips increases in general inflation by many times over, the situation for these families can only worsen.

The Physical, Cultural, and Health Contexts of the Three Cities

We began the study with the expectation that state welfare policies would have very visible and profound impacts on families' lives. The reality of the situation turned out to be much more complex, and differences in the real consequences of state policies were hard to distinguish from other factors related to the labor and housing markets. Massachusetts may have high TANF grants and more generous food stamp and Medicaid policies than Texas, but it also has a tighter housing market and families there must rely on subsidized housing to a greater extent than in San Antonio. Despite its history of more liberal welfare policies, the Massachusetts reforms were, at least on paper, more restrictive in many ways than those adopted in Texas. As part of Massachusetts's reforms, a recipient of TANF can be on the rolls for only two years before being dropped for a year, after which she or he may reapply until the five-year federal limit is reached. In Texas and Illinois, a recipient can remain on TANF for the whole federally mandated five years at a time. During the time of our study, Texas provided many exemptions to the legislated time limits.

The fact that we found few substantial differences among cities no doubt reflects the fact that our families were all at the bottom of the income hierarchy in each city, which meant that they experienced relative, as well as absolute, poverty. Given the stigmatized nature of TANF and other welfare programs in all states, the experiences of poor families are roughly similar, regardless of their state of residence. All of our families were able to find housing, frequently in undesirable neighborhoods and often in substandard housing units. The differences that the city of residence made turned out to be more subtle and reflected aspects of the physical and social environment, the culture, and the weather as much as they did formal policies. In all three cities, however, being poor meant that one did not have the social capital or power to control one's life or that of one's children in important ways. Although families in Massachusetts were better able to obtain and maintain health care coverage, especially for adults, that coverage was still problematic and subject to bureaucratic discontinuities. Although more children in Texas experienced lapses in health coverage than in the two other states, as in Massachusetts and Illinois, most young children in very poor families were eligible for Medicaid and usually received it if their parents conformed to the bureaucratic requirements.

The chapters that follow provide a glimpse into the lives of poor families and reveal the consequences of the lack of a universal health care financing system for poor children and adults in the United States. The stories we recount and the data we present illustrate how the two-tiered system of employment-based comprehensive coverage and Medicare for the middle class and the elderly and the more limited means-tested system of coverage for poor children penalizes families that face the most serious health risks and undermines the productivity of future generations of workers. These stories also reveal the illogic of a system that penalizes individuals' efforts to work and to become self-sufficient. Perhaps most importantly, however, the data clearly reveal that the most serious health risks and the lack of health insurance are not borne equally by all groups. Rather, the negative consequences of poverty, ill health, and inadequate health care take their toll most heavily among minority Americans.

The Structure of What Follows

The first three chapters of this book set the stage for what is to follow. Chapters 2 and 3 provide the background for the more detailed examination of the impact of health care insurance instability on families. In Chapter 2, we review the history of the development of our unique employment-based system of health insurance coverage and delineate the larger policies related to the health care safety net for the poor. In Chapter 3, we review some of the local conditions that affect access to public health insurance and illustrate the sources and nature of the difficulties impoverished families face in obtaining and maintaining health care coverage. In these three chapters, we frame our basic argument that the system of employment-based health care coverage with an ancillary safety net for the poor presents serious challenges to ensuring continuous, high-quality health care for all Americans.

In the second section of this book, Chapters 4, 5, and 6, we draw upon our survey and ethnographic data to examine three sets of factors that influence a family's ability to obtain and maintain health care coverage. In Chapter 4, we examine how families' access to health insurance varies according to the city and state in which they live. In this chapter, we present a more detailed picture of the three cities from the standpoint of families in poverty and summarize state differences in health policies for the poor. In Chapter 5, we examine the tie between employment and health insurance coverage and explain why employment is not a source of health insurance for working poor families. In this chapter, we document the catch-22 that many families find themselves in because of the fact that the less they rely on the welfare system and the more they rely on employment to sustain themselves, the less likely it is that all family members will have health care coverage. In Chapter 6, we deal specifically with the issue of race and ethnicity. African Americans and Hispanics are more likely than non-Hispanic whites to be employed in the sorts of service-sector jobs that do not provide benefits, including health care coverage. Mexican Americans are the least likely to have health insurance of any group in the United States. Although to some extent this reflects the high proportion of Mexican Americans in Texas, the state with the highest number of uninsured citizens in the country, Mexican-origin families are also less likely than non-Hispanic families to have health insurance in both Boston and Chicago.

In the third section of the book, Chapters 7 and 8, we examine the impact of health insurance policy and practice on the lives of children, their parents, and society more generally. In Chapter 7, we review the almost complete lack of health care coverage for low-income adults. Even when parents are able to get Medicaid or SCHIP for their children, they often do without needed care themselves. In Chapter 8, we discuss the future of health care reform in the United States and speculate about the consequences of possible future avenues. In this chapter, we note that although large-scale health care financing reform efforts have historically been unsuccessful in the United States, the drain on the economy and business posed by increasing health care costs, and the fact that more middle-class Americans are paying more for less coverage, will give a new urgency to the need to engage in more than small-scale efforts in the not-too-distant future. As with all reforms, these will have profound implications for poor families.

2

The Health Care Welfare State in America

Sarah, an African American mother of four young children, about whom we will learn more later, did not have medical insurance for herself and had to deal with frequent lapses in her children's coverage. All four children had serious medical problems, and Sarah faced an ongoing struggle to get them the care they needed as well as deal with her own health problems. Three of the children had asthma; the fourth child was born three months prematurely and suffered from lingering respiratory problems. Sarah's work hours and the wages she earned as a staff member at a health care facility varied from week to week, and the children's eligibility for Medicaid changed along with her income. When she was working, Sarah could not afford to take the time off for the recertification visits that were required to maintain each child's Medicaid. In order to take the children to the doctor, Sarah had to take even more time off from work, which she could hardly afford. She was not paid for the hours she took off and, like many other marginal workers, she risked getting fired if she was absent too often.

Sarah's experiences in obtaining health care for her children were typical of those of the low-income mothers we interviewed and illustrate the ways in which the instability of household health insurance relates directly to instability in work, child care, transportation, and a parent's own health problems. We found that because of the complexity and interconnectedness of the problems that poor families face, rarely did one problem stand out as primary. They occurred in combination and easily overwhelmed a family's social and limited economic resources. We return to this theme throughout the book. Although our focus is on health and health insurance, other problem areas are intimately intertwined with health issues, and all of these problems work together to create the instability with which Sarah and other low-income parents must continuously grapple.

Sarah's ability to get her children the medical care they needed was made more difficult by the fact that she had no car and getting the children to the doctor was complicated and time-consuming. The need to use public transportation, which involved waiting for buses and in many cases the need to make more than one transfer, transformed what might have been a two-hour undertaking if she had owned a car into an all-day affair. As a result, Sarah avoided doctor visits for the children unless there was a clear medical problem. As she told us, "I just take them when they need it [or for their inoculations]. I really don't do the checkup thing like I'm supposed to, but I take them when they're sick or I see something that's not going right." Although she was able to maintain Medicaid coverage for her children at least some of the time, Sarah herself had no health insurance. Her dilemma was a common one among our respondents. Her job offered no benefits, yet she was not eligible for Medicaid. Like so many of the other mothers we interviewed, she did not know what she would do if she were to become seriously ill and need medical care.

Sarah's dilemma reflects basic structural problems in the way that health care for the poor is provided in the United States. As in other developed nations, health care policy in the United States represents a core component of welfare and labor policy more generally, and also as in other nations, U.S. welfare policy reflects basic aspects of the nation's political and economic history (Hicks 1999; Huber and Stephens 2001a; Huber and Stephens 2001b; Quadagno 2004). The partial nature of public health care coverage in the United States, as illustrated by Sarah's situation, is matched by the partial nature of other welfare services and reflects a political economy in which government control of the job market and worker benefits is relatively limited and in which labor unions have been rather ineffective in furthering a national welfare agenda that includes public health care coverage (Asher and Stephenson 1990; Esping-Andersen 1990; Esping-Andersen 1999; Hoffman 2001; King and Wood 1999; Quadagno 2005; Starr 1982; Weir, Orloff, and Skocpol 1988). Understanding U.S. health care financing policy, with its heavy reliance on employer-based insurance, as well as the impact of that policy on low-income families requires attention to the broader policy picture within which the U.S. health care system has evolved. Such an examination allows us to identify the major roadblocks to system reform. It also enables us to more fully understand the possible responses by federal and state governments to the extraordinary growth in health care costs at a time of decreasing public revenues and increasing budgetary constraints.

Health Care in the United States: Two Incomplete Systems

In the United States, most health care for families and children is financed from two sources: private insurance that consists primarily of group policies provided by employers, and programs sponsored by the government. Since Medicare and Medicaid were introduced in 1965, a growing share of health care costs has been paid by federal and state governments rather than by individual patients or private insurers. Although most middle-class Americans are still covered by private employer-based plans, the proportion of Americans covered by private insurance is decreasing (U.S. Bureau of the Census 2005). As medical care inflation drives the cost of health care plans ever higher, a growing number of employers are not offering coverage to their employees or requiring employees to pay larger premiums to offset the cost of such policies, leading a growing number of employees not to participate (Long and Shen 2004). Although the decline in employer-sponsored health insurance has been driven to a large extent by economics, it also reflects a longer-term weakening of organized labor and an overt hostility by employers to unionization and workers' rights generally (Tilly 2004). Even Europe, with its far more comprehensive social welfare net and generous public health policies, faces challenges in maintaining that system intact in the face of globalized economic competition (Koivusalo 2005).

A summary of recent trends in sources of health care coverage compiled by *Child Trends* illustrates this shift in coverage for children in the United States. Between 2000 and 2003, the percentage of all children under eighteen with private health insurance coverage decreased from 71 percent to 66 percent. At the same time, the percentage of children enrolled in Medicaid increased from 20 percent to 26 percent

(Child Trends Data Bank 2003). The fundamental systemic problem that we are facing, however, arises from the fact that a large fraction of children fall through the cracks and are not covered by either system (Dubay, Haley, and Kenney 2002; Guyer 2000; Perry et al. 2000). In addition, for reasons we will explore later, a large number of children who qualify for Medicaid and SCHIP on the basis of their family's income do not participate (Hill and Lutzky 2003).

Part of the increase in the number of the uninsured can be attributed to the fact that a growing proportion of workers are employed in jobs that do not offer health care coverage (Long and Shen 2004; Shen and Zuckerman 2003). In recent years, the proportion of workers employed in services has increased at the same time that employment in manufacturing has decreased. In addition, a growing fraction of workers are working part-time or for small firms that do not have the employee base to negotiate favorable group health plans (Long and Shen 2004). Although these changes affect all groups and are increasing the employment and social benefit insecurity of a large fraction of Americans, they affect certain subgroups disproportionately. Many of these marginal workers are African American and Hispanic and have low levels of education and few job skills. One particularly vulnerable group, which many would exclude from the receipt of social services altogether, are noncitizens and their children (Chollet 1994). We will deal with the impact of these trends in employment and with the particular vulnerabilities of African and Hispanic Americans in greater detail in subsequent chapters.

One of the major failures of our current health care system generally that became tragically apparent in the Three City Study is the fact that it offers almost no options for health care coverage for working poor adults. Without access to an employer-sponsored group health plan that can be purchased for a reasonable price, even working adults with incomes well above the poverty line cannot afford to purchase private coverage. Only a handful of our respondents had access to affordable health insurance on a long-term basis. Some were able to maintain coverage for short periods, but these periods were frequently interrupted by periods during which they had no coverage. Like Sarah, many adults who work even full-time have no choice but to neglect their health and focus on doing what they can for their children. As we will see in subsequent chapters, many poor families accumulate massive medical debt that they can never realistically pay off and that becomes a serious economic burden and a barrier to getting ahead.

A Limited Welfare State

In the literature on the welfare state, the United States is characterized as an outlier because of the relatively limited role that the state plays in providing the full range of social services to its citizens (Esping-Andersen 1990; Esping-Andersen 1999; Hicks 1999; Noble 1997; Wier, Orloff, and Skocpol 1988). Unlike the citizens of Europe, Americans do not receive, and for the most part do not expect, free higher education, state-mandated vacations, family allowances, or guaranteed health care as basic citizenship rights. For most of those over sixty-five, Social Security and Medicare provide income support and universal health coverage, but for younger individuals no such universal programs exist. Except for the poorest Americans, or those with disabilities or certain serious health problems, basic services must be purchased on the open market or paid for by privately purchased or employer-sponsored health insurance.

An exclusive focus on public expenditures for social welfare, however, especially on programs directed to the poor, can be quite misleading and seriously underestimate the total amount of national income that is devoted to social welfare broadly defined. Since the late 1980s, several observers have pointed out that real social welfare expenditures in the United States are every bit as high as they are in the more developed welfare states of Europe; they simply appear in a different part of the national ledger (Gilbert and Gilbert 1989; Gottschalk 2000; Hacker 2002; Howard 1997; Stevens 1988). In the United States, tax incentives for pension and health plans, credit subsidies, and other indirect transfers account for a major component of aggregate expenditures for social welfare, paid for publicly in terms of forgone tax revenues (Hacker 2002). Social Security and Medicare, tax exemptions for employers and employees for health insurance and pension plans, and other publicly subsidized private benefits for the middle class represent major direct and indirect investments in social welfare.

Yet the fact that a large fraction of total social spending in the United States is indirect and subsidizes benefits for the middle class has a major distributional impact, as well as important implications for the health and welfare of the poor. As Jacob S. Hacker notes, "It matters fundamentally whether a nation's social welfare framework is characterized by low public spending, low taxes, and high private spending, on the one hand, or high public spending, high taxes, and low private spending, on the other; and this is true even if after-tax spending is identical" (Hacker 2002, p. 23). In the first scenario, characteristic of the United States, the beneficiaries are disproportionately the middle and upper classes, whereas in the second scenario, typical of the more extensive welfare states of Europe, benefits are more equally distributed and the lower classes benefit to a much larger extent. These more egalitarian societies are characterized by far less income inequality and lower rates of poverty than in the United States (Smeeding 2000; Smeeding, Rainwater, and Burtless 2001). Clearly, these different social welfare systems and philosophies for providing public goods can result in profound class-based disparities in health.

Of course, even in a free-market-based open economy, the state plays a major role in regulating interstate commerce, ensuring product safety, overseeing securities markets, and regulating much of collective life, including the health care industry. Yet, in the United States, the state's intrusion into the market, and especially into the area of labor relations and economic rights, remains far below that typical of Europe (Hacker 2002; King and Wood 1999). The social democratic or Christian democratic traditions of Europe and the class-based social structures typical of many of the developed welfare states are foreign to the United States, where labor has been unsupportive of, and at times even hostile to, universal health care (Hoffman 2001; Numbers 1978; Quadagno 2005; Starr 1982). In the United States, the level of intrusion by the state into labor–management relations typical of some other nations would be intolerable. In this country, if an employer offers a retirement plan to its employees, specific statutes dictate its content and vesting. If the employer offers a health plan, the law also specifies what that plan must cover, depending upon whether the employer self-insures or purchases the coverage from a third party. Employers, however, are not required to offer retirement or health plans to their employees, and they can withdraw coverage pretty much as they wish. If a firm can attract the workers it needs without such benefits, only a highly developed sense of social responsibility would motivate it to do so. Nor does the state seriously restrict an employer's right to fire employees. In the absence of a strong Labor Party, labor relations and the benefits that employees receive in the United States are dictated largely by economic efficiency and the labor needs of employers. In a market economy with employer-sponsored private benefits, the continuity of those benefits over the long term also depends to a large degree on the tightness or looseness of the labor market.

The extent to which labor market freedom and the absence of an extensive welfare state account for the remarkable ability of the U.S. economy to produce wealth is unclear. Those opposed to high levels of spending on social programs point out that universal and comprehensive social welfare entitlements require high marginal tax rates that can divert capital from production to consumption (Flora 1986). Additionally, social programs very quickly become entitlements and create expectations that make it difficult for governments to adapt to fiscal crises and to reduce social expenditures in order to deal with such crises (Bonoli 2001; Marmor, Mashaw, and Harvey 1990; Stephens 1996). Even at a time during which they face serious economic challenges that might call for reducing social welfare expenditures, European welfare states find it difficult to do so (Koivusalo 2005; Pierson 1994a; Scarborough 2000). Nonetheless, since the 1970s, all developed nations have experienced at least some retrenchment, or at least a slowing of the increase in their expenditures on welfare. These changes are the result of globalization and the worldwide economic crises that began after the abandonment of the Bretton Woods system of international fixed currency-exchange rates and the petroleum supply crisis spawned by OPEC price increases (Kitschelt et al. 1999; Stephens, Huber, and Ray 1999; Swank 2001). Other structural and demographic forces, including the shift from manufacturing to service employment and the rapid aging of the populations of the developed nations, are placing increasing economic strains on modern welfare states. These changes reduce economic growth rates at the same time that they increase expenditures for pensions and health care (Pierson 2001b).

Yet many European nations have maintained dynamic economies and high rates of productivity while extending publicly financed universal and comprehensive citizenship entitlements (Esping-Andersen 1990; Esping-Andersen 1999). It is clear that investments in people can increase productivity as effectively as investments in capital and that there is no inherent conflict between investments in workers and

investments in material capital. Indeed, such investments are comple-
mentary (Esping-Andersen et al. 2002; Katz 2001). The welfare state
involves more than just the redistribution of wealth. In addition to
increasing worker productivity, a paternalistic state can foster a sense
of citizenship, belonging, and participation that a purely competitive
market-based system can undermine.

Over half a century ago, T. H. Marshall (Marshall 1950) conceptu-
alized the modern welfare state as the culmination of three centuries
of consolidation of basic human rights that define full citizenship.
According to Marshall, the process began in the eighteenth century
with guarantees of legal and civil rights, progressed in the nineteenth
century with the extension of political rights, and reached its logical
culmination with the twentieth century's struggles for social rights,
including full participation in the economy and the right to the material necessities of a civilized and productive life. Today, many groups
in the developing world are characterized by what has been termed
"low-intensity citizenship," a phrase that emphasizes their incomplete
incorporation into the body politic or the economy. Many of these
individuals are indigenous peoples or racial and ethnic minorities, as
we shall discuss in the context of the United States. Clearly, Marshall's
third stage, the realization of the full range of human rights, remains
incomplete in many parts of the world, and it is only partially complete in the United States. The completion of the third stage, as well as
earlier stages, requires a change in political consciousness. Although
Social Security, Medicare, and programs for the poorest citizens are
widely accepted by Americans, universal health care and the other
social guarantees typical of advanced welfare states remain foreign to
our political consciousness. Yet the demographic, economic, and social
changes that we witnessed during the latter half of the twentieth century will require a new approach to the definition of citizenship and the
guarantee of basic human rights. Understanding what those changes
will be, using health insurance as our key example, and identifying the
forces that will bring them about forms the core motivation for our
discussion.

The specific nature of each nation's welfare state clearly reflects local
historical, economic, political, and cultural factors, as well as more
global forces. Esping-Andersen's (1990) three-part typology of welfare states captures some of that reality. The Nordic model, typified

by Sweden, Norway, and Denmark, includes comprehensive and universal coverage of the full range of services from education to family support financed largely by high taxes. The Central European model evolved along more corporatist or class-based lines, with generous benefits closely tied to union membership and labor-sector affiliations (Esping-Andersen 1990; Esping-Andersen 1999; Golden, Wallerstein, and Lange 1999). Southern Europe and nations such as Japan continue to look toward the family to care for aging parents and provide other social supports while providing some nationalized services such as child care. Yet the global economic situation has worsened and the golden age of the welfare state may be permanently over. Globalization has undermined the ability of nations to isolate their economies from international competition, and the world as a whole may be forced to learn to live with permanent austerity (Pierson 2001a). This period of austerity has arrived before many nations of the developing world have attained the capacity to provide even basic social services to large segments of their populations. It has also arrived at a time when the welfare state in the United States is incomplete and political forces are seeking its retrenchment.

Regardless of their level of development, each welfare state is forced to deal with a core set of problems that include old-age security and health care. During the closing decades of the twentieth century, aging populations, the easy transmission of diseases across the globe, and the explosive growth in the cost of modern medicine presented monumental fiscal challenges worldwide. These will only increase as we move into the new century. In this new world, equity in the distribution of health care across social classes becomes even more difficult to guarantee. For example, although enrollment in the new State Children's Health Insurance Program (SCHIP) grew rapidly during the first six years of its existence, in 2003 enrollment slowed as states grappled with a new fiscal austerity (Dunkelberg and O'Malley 2004; Smith and Rousseau 2003; Smith, Rousseau, and O'Malley 2004; Smith et al. 2004). The Sudden Acute Respiratory Syndrome (SARS) outbreaks in Asia and the well-established global HIV/AIDS pandemic are probably only the beginning of what we will witness as part of the globalization of diseases and other health care challenges. In the developed world, an epidemic of obesity and the costs of treatments for the chronic conditions of aging will continue to add to already soaring health care costs. As the population ages, long-term care will consume an ever larger share of public budgets (Kaiser Commission 2004). Issues of rationing, equity, and efficiency in health care will be with us for many years as the role of medicine in our lives increases. Permanent austerity presents particularly serious problems for poor families such as those in our study, who could easily find that they are the big losers in any attempt to contain costs.

The Redistributional Aspects of Health Care

Unless a health care system is completely market-based, and we can think of none that is, it will have some redistributional characteristics because publicly financed care, even at low levels, represents a transfer to the poor. Optimal population health and well-being simply cannot be achieved in the presence of high levels of inequality in income and wealth, particularly when material resources determine access to health care. Historically, inequalities in wealth have manifested themselves as inequalities in morbidity and mortality (Link and Phelan 1995). If poverty and its serious physical, social, and emotional health consequences are to be overcome, some level of effective income redistribution, or at least the ability to access the things that money can buy, including health care, is necessary.

Regardless of how one measures it, poverty in the United States, especially for minority children, is far higher than that of other developed nations, even those with much lower average incomes (Smeeding, Rainwater, and Burtless 2001). What is perhaps more disturbing, not least because of its potential impact on health, is the degree of relative poverty between those at the lowest end of the income distribution and those at the highest end. Those in the lowest tenth of the income distribution make only 34 to 38 percent of the median U.S. income (Gottschalk and Smeeding 2000; Smeeding 2000). The United States has a higher proportion of very low-paying jobs than is the case in other developed nations (Smeeding, Rainwater, and Burtless 2001). In other countries, social spending, which reduces the poverty rate, especially for families with children, compensates for low wages. In the United States, low levels of social spending leave a growing chasm between the poor and the more affluent in terms of income and such necessities as health care.

As we shall discuss in later chapters, because African Americans and Latinos are disproportionately poor, they bear the greatest burden of illness and have the least secure access to health insurance and health care. The brunt of these differences is borne in large part by children in impoverished families, who face a particularly high likelihood of spending part of their childhood in poverty. There is continuing evidence that children in poverty not only experience lapses in health insurance but also experience exposure to health risks related to the neighborhoods in which they live and the lapses in medical care they experience.

Not everyone finds high levels of inequality to be bad, however. More than a century after Yale sociologist and political theorist William Graham Sumner (Sumner 1883) preached the gospel of social Darwinism, with the message that inequality is the result of a natural economic order and that any attempt to eliminate poverty would result in disaster, inequality is still with us, as is the point of view that it is not only inevitable but functional. Even today, some hold that inequality provides incentives for individuals to strive to better their lot in life and ultimately contributes to an overall economic efficiency that improves the situation even of those at the bottom of the economic hierarchy (Welch 1999). The answer to the question of whether extreme inequality is good or even tolerable, however, does not hinge on technical considerations but rather on profoundly ethical choices that ultimately reflect a society's moral character. There can be little doubt that the scourge of hunger motivates people to accept employment or tasks that they would otherwise reject, but most modern societies have turned away from reward systems based on serious deprivation.

Of course, apologists for the level of inequality that we experience in the United States would say that the consequences of the level of inequality we experience are not that bad and that the objective situation of the poor in any developed nation is far better than that of the poor in the developing world or those of previous historical periods. For the most part, the poor have shelter, receive charity health care for acute problems, and often own cars. Although in an absolute sense the poor in the United States are indeed better off today than in earlier eras or than the poor in many developing nations today, one must still question the justice of such inequality. Despite the claim that inequality contributes to economic efficiency, inequality is not part of a process that leads to its own elimination. Inequality and poverty in the United States have remained remarkably intransigent despite high levels of economic growth that have benefited those who are better-off but left those at the bottom, or at least a good number of them, pretty much where they were. Although many of the poorest Americans benefited from the economic boom of the 1990s, it is clear that economic growth alone cannot eliminate poverty (Freeman 2001). The inevitable economic slowdowns that follow boom periods erode even the modest employment and income gains that the poor are able to make. They are always the last hired and first fired, and they are often employed in jobs that hang by an economic thread. Even in economic booms, we retain a stratum of jobs that keeps the working poor who depend on them unstably employed and at high risk of poverty.

Health and the Equality of Opportunity

From affirmative action to social welfare, Americans value equality of opportunity and reject equality of outcomes. Yet a careful examination of the nature of work and the system of social stratification in the United States, especially as they affect minority-group members, makes it clear that equality of opportunity as distinct from equality of outcomes is a myth. The focus on equality of opportunity allows us to avoid difficult questions of equity and fairness in real access to social goods. It is hard to imagine that anyone would claim that a social system guarantees equality of opportunity if its health care system increases the risk of premature birth and lifelong impairments for certain of its citizens. Similarly, because productivity and the possibility of social mobility depend on good health and vitality, a system that provides high-quality health care to the middle class but lower-quality care to working-class and minority households does not provide equality of opportunity. When it comes to education, health care, and those human capital inputs that are essential to economic success, equality of access to services, particularly for children, is the only way to guarantee equality of opportunity.

In the United States, opportunities in education, the labor market, and health care have been greatly influenced by a history of slavery and racism that has left us with a disproportionate fraction of the poor who are black and Hispanic (Gilens 1999; Quadagno 1994; Weir, Orloff, and Skocpol 1988). Structural factors interact with ascribed characteristics to determine both the risk of poor health and one's access to health care. Even in the midst of growing post–World War II prosperity, large segments of the population benefited only minimally and were left behind economically. Again, these individuals were disproportionately black and Hispanic. Poverty, of course, does not respect skin color, and the majority of the poor are non-Hispanic and white simply because non-Hispanic whites make up a large majority of the population. There can be little doubt, however, that in the United States race has directly and profoundly influenced the politics of social welfare (Goodwin 1997; Lieberman 1998; Mink 1995; Mink 1998; O'Connor 2001; Piven 1971; Weir, Orloff, and Skocpol 1988).

The New Reality of Work: Contingency and the Lack of Benefits

The literature on the welfare state draws heavily on the concept of "path dependence," which refers to the fact that once institutions or institutionalized practices are in place, they create constituencies and organizational actors with stakes in the status quo (Pierson 1994b). Organizations and their missions are hard to change because administrators, bureaucrats, employees, and clients resist change for any number of reasons. Institutional inertia is a simple fact of organizational life. Even conservative governments in the highly developed welfare states of Europe find it difficult to change health, pension, and other benefit programs because of intense resistance from their beneficiaries. Conversely, advocates for the poor in the more liberal welfare states find that attempts to extend welfare programs run into the vociferous resistance of conservatives, business representatives, and other interested groups. President Bill Clinton's health insurance plan drew withering opposition from the insurance industry and other parties that have deep stakes in the status quo. That opposition, as in the case of all previous attempts at radical change in our health insurance system, doomed the Clinton plan (Daniels, Light, and Caplan 1996; Skocpol 1996; Starr 1994).

Yet organizations and government policies do change, usually slowly but sometimes rapidly, in response to crises. In a relatively short period, health care financing in the United States shifted from a fee-for-service system based on usual and customary fees to a managed-care arrangement with predetermined budgets despite the strong opposition of the American Medical Association and other interested parties (Starr 1982). The rise in health care costs remains a motivation for change, but to date the changes experienced in the United States still leave a significant part of the population uninsured and often lacking regular health care, as well as many who are insured but with less coverage and greater out-of-pocket expenditures.

In fact, one consequence of the rapid and apparently endless rise in the cost of health care is that more of the middle class find that they face the health care uncertainties and precariousness long experienced by the working class (Sullivan, Warren, and Westbrook 2000). Early retirees and even those who qualify for Medicare find themselves without the supplemental coverage or income they need to pay for prescription drugs or other medical services (Weller, Wenger, and Gould 2004). Globalization and market uncertainties create the need for a highly flexible labor force that allows firms to react quickly to changing situations. Contingent employment, outsourcing, and just-in-time inventorying increasingly create an employment environment in which the tie between employer and employee has loosened and become less paternalistic (Belous 1989; Polivka 1989; Schultze 2000; Spalter-Roth and Hartman 1998). Although certain high-productivity workers must be kept on the payroll even in slow economic times to ensure that they will be available when economic activity picks up, production line workers, office staff, and maintenance workers are only needed on a contingent basis.

Increasingly, rather than maintaining their own staffs to carry out routine administrative or production functions, employers purchase these services from independent contractors (Barker and Christensen 1998). Many long-time traditional employees are shifted to the role of independent contractor with no formal tie to the employer. By contracting out routine tasks, the firm is no longer responsible for providing benefits to the employees who perform these tasks. As the cost of health insurance rises and as employers find that they cannot shift the increased cost onto employees, the logical business response is to reduce the number of employees and purchase those services rather than provide them in-house. In such a system of contingent work, many more individuals will inevitably find themselves without benefits or in the position of having to buy expensive private policies. Without the guarantees of a group plan, many will find that preexisting conditions, high cost, and other barriers will leave them without adequate individual or family coverage. As more of the population finds itself experiencing the health care uncertainties that the poor have lived with for decades, the funding, organization, and reach of public health care will experience more pressure to change.

This book provides insight into the health care vulnerabilities of the poor under our current system and suggests ways in which a new system might benefit not only them but also the new contingent working class. In this new work environment, the incomes of the poorest workers continue to decline, in large part because of their relative lack of skills (Autor, Katz, and Kearny 2005). Although observers from different points to the left or right of the political spectrum disagree on whether inequality itself is a problem and in the solutions they offer to the deteriorating situation of the working poor, few deny that the worsening situation of those at the bottom of the economic hierarchy has serious long-term implications for individuals and society at large (Ellwood et al. 2000). The low-skill African Americans and Hispanics who participated in our study find themselves in the most precarious position.

Health Care and the Common Weal

The point we make is fairly simple: Our system of employment-based health insurance coverage does not work for poor families, especially those dependent on low-wage jobs, nor does it address the needs of a large fraction of minority Americans. Given improved health levels and progress in medical care, what constitutes a minimal level of health is far higher today than it might have been in previous centuries or even earlier decades of this century. In a world in which everyone's health and vitality were compromised and in which healers had only an herbal pharmacopoeia and relatively inexpensive and largely ineffective palliatives to offer, perhaps something close to self-sufficiency in health care was possible. Today, a common chronic health problem or a serious acute illness can result in expenditures that are beyond the ability of all but the wealthiest families to bear. As health levels have improved and the possibility of treating problems has evolved, the poor health and bad teeth that were common in previous decades have become intolerable.

Certainly, avoidable and correctable differences in health and vitality are unfair in and of themselves, but we need not call solely upon
altruism or an abstract sense of social justice to make the case for a
more comprehensive and equitable health care system. The core reality
of our collective social life is that everyone's welfare will at some point
depend upon the health and productive capacity of others. Our rapidly
aging and retired population must be supported by the contributions of
those still in the labor force. At the same time, the schools that educate
future workers, like every other public institution, depend entirely on
the wealth created by those who are currently employed. The problem we face and our dependence on a growing minority workforce are
dramatically illustrated by Social Security. In 1945, a decade after the
program was introduced, there were approximately forty workers contributing to the support of each retired worker. By 2003, that number
had shrunk to slightly more than three, and by 2030 only two workers will contribute to the support of each retired baby boomer (Social
Security Administration 2004a). Whether or not one believes that there
is a fundamental flaw in the way Social Security is funded, there can
be little doubt that if the program remains a pay-as-you-go system in
which the support of the retired population comes directly from the
paychecks of those who are still working, each employed American
will have to contribute a large fraction of his or her income in Social
Security and Medicare taxes (Bongaarts 2004).

The potential problem is again made more serious by the fact that
the high growth rates and the relative youth of the African American
and Hispanic populations mean that the workforce of the future will
become increasingly minority. If the productivity of these minority
workers is compromised by low educational levels or poor health, the
productive potential of the economy as a whole will be placed in serious
jeopardy. In the chapters that follow, we will reveal the conditions in
which a large segment of the future labor force is spending its childhood
and adolescence. These conditions are not conducive to the development of the highest levels of physical, emotional, or social health. As we
will show, the health risks that these future workers face are the result
of structural factors related to the labor market in which their parents find employment and the incomplete nature of the social welfare
safety net that guarantees their health and welfare. Those children who
today suffer serious educational and other disadvantages, and who will

as a consequence find themselves restricted to low-wage occupations in adulthood, will not have the resources, nor will they likely be willing, to shoulder the burden of supporting a disproportionately non-Hispanic white elderly population (Angel and Angel 2005; Lee 1997). This racial and ethnic overlay lends a potentially explosive dimension to the crisis of having to support an aging retired population at the same time that our nation will face new challenges in the war on terror, the education of the young, the decay of our metropolitan areas, and serious global economic competition.

The history, organization, and financing of health care in the United States that we have briefly outlined in this chapter are fairly well known. What is less well understood are the consequences of that system for the most vulnerable Americans. Since the introduction of Medicare in 1965, elderly Americans have benefited from universal, although incomplete, coverage. For the poor, and especially children and pregnant women, Medicaid and the State Children's Health Insurance Program (SCHIP) provide a safety net and access to basic care, although in 2003 enrollment in this vital program declined in response to the new fiscal crisis (Dunkelberg and O'Malley 2004; Smith, Rousseau, and O'Malley 2004). Again we encounter inequities based on race and ethnicity. One of the most disturbing aspects of our health care financing system that the Three City Study underscores is the extent to which rates of Medicaid coverage vary among racial and ethnic groups. As we demonstrate, rates of health insurance coverage among Mexican Americans are shockingly low. Our data, as well as many other studies, also reveal important differences in coverage between single-parent and couple-headed families that are a direct consequence of policies that penalize marriage despite the stated desire of policymakers to strengthen the family (Wheaton 1998).

Health forms the basis of individual well-being and contributes to general public prosperity. Unhealthy children become unhealthy adults, and for that reason the focus of the limited means-tested health care system we have has always focused primarily on children. Since the introduction of Medicaid, the recognition of the importance of adequate preventive and acute care in childhood has resulted in initiatives at both the federal and state levels to extend coverage to more children at older ages, even in families with incomes above the poverty level. These initiatives are clearly significant and needed extensions of

a vital governmental function. The families in our studies clearly benefited from and appreciated the fact that they could at least get publicly
funded coverage for their children. As we will see, almost all families
valued Medicaid highly. Yet our system of health care financing remains
very incomplete, especially for medically needy adults and the working
poor. As we document, even in families with incomes low enough to
qualify for Medicaid, many children are not enrolled. Ultimately, our
study leads us to the conclusion that in order to address these shortcomings more central coordination of the entire health care delivery
system will be necessary even if the centralization and bureaucracy it
requires goes against our historical preferences. We end the book with
a discussion of the possibilities.

The three cities in our study revealed certain common patterns in
health care coverage among low-income families, such as a lower probability of Medicaid coverage the longer a family has been off the cash
assistance rolls. Yet there were important differences among the families we interviewed. Some poor families and even some that left the
cash assistance rolls managed to obtain employer-sponsored coverage
at least sporadically. These were a very small minority, however, and
it is clear from our research that for families on welfare employment
is rarely a route to self-sufficiency in income or health care coverage.
Most heads of households in our study were employed irregularly.
Very few had a career or even what we might consider a steady job.
The question we then must ask is what those without Medicaid or
employer-based coverage do for health care. The findings from the
ethnography suggest that they patch together services from different
sources for different problems, accumulate debt, do without care, or
resort to a combination of all of these. The result is a lack of continuity
of care and potentially lower-quality care.

Our purpose in comparing the situations of poor families in three
cities in states with different political, economic, and social histories
was to determine how much of a difference local welfare policy and
its implementation make in the lives of poor families. Massachusetts is
a much more liberal state than Texas, where the introduction of even
a modest income tax has been impossible and in which spending on
welfare has traditionally been low. Yet when it comes to TANF, as
we noted earlier, Massachusetts has what on paper looks like a more
punitive and restrictive policy than Texas. In Massachusetts, one can

receive TANF continuously only for a two-year period before being forced off at least for awhile. Understanding the barriers that face impoverished families who find themselves periodically dependent on welfare is complicated by the nature of the regulatory system in most states. Texas has many exemptions for the mothers of young children and others, as do Massachusetts and Illinois. All states have a complex set of sanctions that they impose on TANF recipients that can easily result in their losing benefits, at least temporarily, for noncompliance with TANF rules and regulations. Although state and local differences, which we discuss in Chapter 4, as well as the differential availability of medical care, housing, and transportation, can have a significant impact on a family's access to services, our ethnographic interviews show that the basic problems of poverty are common to all sites and largely reflect the way in which welfare policy is determined in Washington. The problems of the poor arise from their tenuous tie to the labor market and the fact that very few are able to greatly improve their lot through work alone. Because the labor market is the source not only of income but of health and retirement benefits, despite the generosity of state or local welfare policies those at the bottom of the occupational hierarchy who cycle between work and unemployment find it difficult to get ahead and particularly difficult to maintain regular health insurance for all family members, no matter where they live. In what follows, we illustrate the health-related impact of this complex nexus of work, family, and social policy on individual families as their lives unfolded during the time we were in contact with them. We begin in the next chapter by exploring the differences among the three cities as settings for the search for social services and health care by low-income families.

Health Insurance as a Social Marker

In the end, participation in Medicaid and other health-related programs serves as an indicator of a family's degree of incorporation into social life generally. Families without complete family coverage are not only at risk of poor health and medical indebtedness but also lack an important marker of full citizenship. Without the material basis of a stable and productive life, to which adequate health care is central, full participation in civic and economic life is not possible. Such families lack an important component of what makes up the social rights that we mentioned earlier in the chapter (Marshall 1950). As surveys and administrative data show, and as our ethnographic data make tragically clear, those families with incomplete health care coverage almost inevitably find themselves mired in a situation in which they must struggle, often unsuccessfully, to achieve basic security. The struggle for health care coverage is only a component of the overall battle. The families we studied had little access to stable employment with stable wages that might move them out of poverty. Many were forced to move frequently in search of less expensive or subsidized housing. Such residential instability often made it difficult for us to maintain contact with the families in our study, and it certainly added to the instability of their lives. These families rarely had easy or dependable access to transportation to work, to school, or to health care facilities. Although the centerpiece of our analysis is health care insurance, from the perspective of the families we studied, health insurance is just one strand in a tangle of problems that resulted in continuing instability in family life. In the next chapter, we begin to understand how the illogical and incomprehensible system of health care for the poor fails to protect the health of the most vulnerable.

3

The Tattered Health Care Safety Net
for Poor Americans

When we met Claudia, a Latina in her late twenties, she was pregnant with her fifth child and had recently separated from her partner. Like so many of the mothers we interviewed, Claudia was engaged in a nearly constant struggle with the welfare bureaucracy over her family's health coverage. The task was made more difficult by the fact that each of her four boys had to qualify for various social services, including Medicaid, separately and because of their different ages according to different criteria. The fact that family coverage was not available to them presented Claudia, as well as the other families we studied, with a wide range of difficulties. Obviously frustrated, Claudia told us about the problems she encountered in trying to comply with the paperwork requirements for Medicaid and other social welfare programs. Despite her best efforts, often one or another of her children was without health coverage. As she explained,

When I was pregnant, the clinic told me about the Medicaid. So automatically, when I went for the Medicaid, they told me did I need assistance with money for his diapers and stuff, so I went ahead and applied for it.... They had me going crazy, they ask for so many things.... They want a letter from a neighbor or friend stating who lives in your house, and then they want your proof of income, and they want [to know] how many kids are living in your house, and say somebody comes to stay with you, they want to know who comes to stay with you. They're nosy! They're very nosy, things that it doesn't even make sense why they want to know it, but they want to know it.

Even when she thought she had complied with the bureaucratic requirements, however, it was not always enough. Frequent misunderstandings and miscommunication concerning required paperwork and the complicated application and recertification processes resulted in frequent lapses in essential program coverage. Claudia told us of one recent experience:

Like this last time, I just went to renew my food stamps last month. I had already taken them my application. I had already taken them the domicile letter. I took them everything they needed. Then they wrote me that only my seven-year-old was eligible for Medicaid because they didn't have enough information on the rest of the children and they couldn't help me with my food stamps for this month because they didn't have the domicile letter and all the information they needed. I was like, "I already took you the letter – every paper you needed, I took it already, I was ahead of you all." Well, they misplaced everything, so I had to go redo everything all over again.

Although Claudia's particular situation may have been somewhat more complicated than those of other families because she had more children than most of the mothers we interviewed, her story is not all that different from those of the other families, and it illustrates the fact that the health care safety net for poor Americans is far from comprehensive or seamless. For many, if not most, impoverished families in the United States, health care coverage is difficult to obtain, temporary, and inadequate (Angel et al. 2001; Institute of Medicine 2004; Mullahy and Wolfe 2001; Williams et al. 2004). Many low-income families alternate among the often costly plans sometimes available to them through employment, periods without health insurance, and dependence on publicly funded health insurance for at least some members of the family. Of course, in the United States, the poor do not go completely without medical care. The poorest families and those with unemployed parents have access to Medicaid and SCHIP as well as other state-sponsored programs (Cunningham 2003; Hoadley, Cunningham, and McHugh 2004; Reschovsky and Cunningham 1998). Among the unemployed and the poorest working families, these programs largely compensate for the lack of employer-sponsored insurance for children, although even when the children in a family receive Medicaid or SCHIP, the adults often remain uninsured (Blumberg and Holahan 2004a; Blumberg and Holahan 2004b; Long and Shen 2004). Those low-income families that do not qualify for Medicaid or SCHIP often receive free or low-cost care in emergency rooms or charitable clinics (Cornelius 1993; Lillie-Blanton, Leigh, and Alfaro-Correa 1996; Radzwill 2003; Shah-Canning, Alpert, and Bauchner 1996; Thompson and Glick 1999).

Neither Medicaid nor any other program provides complete coverage to all poor children and adults, nor do low-income families enjoy the continuity of coverage and access to care that middle-class Americans take for granted (Freeman et al. 1990; Institute of Medicine 2001; Mullahy and Wolfe 2001; Wolfe and Vanness 1999). At the bottom of our social hierarchy, and increasingly among the working class, health care coverage is prohibitively expensive or simply unavailable for considerable periods of a person's life (Blumberg and Holahan 2004a; Cooper and Schone 1997; Farber and Levy 2000; Gabel et al. 2003; Long and Shen 2004).

The lack of health insurance is part of the pervasive uncertainty and instability of life at the economic margin. Although most middle-class families can budget for routine health expenditures and count on employer-based insurance to cover potentially catastrophic health care expenditures, the poor simply cannot protect themselves against unpredictable events, including illness or accident. Catastrophic medical expenses are one of the leading causes of bankruptcy even for families with substantial resources (Himmelstein et al. 2005; Jacoby, Sullivan, and Warren, 2000; Sullivan, Warren, and Westbrook 2000). Yet, for the poor, the unpredictable and the catastrophic are everyday realities, and their need for health care is often urgent. The poor suffer more physical and mental illnesses and disabling conditions than the more affluent (Blackwell, Hayward, and Crimmins 2001; Burton and Whitfield 2003; Danziger et al. 2000; Geronimus 1996; Heymann 2000; Williams and Collins 1995). Poor health is part of a vicious cycle in which absences from employment because of illness often result in the loss of a job and any possibility of employment-based insurance, thereby contributing to the poverty and insecurity that undermine one's health in the first place (Danziger et al. 2000; Jayakody, Danziger, and Pollack 2000; Repetti, Matthews, and Waldron 1989; Singer and Ryff 2001).

Because they often find it impossible to maintain a regular work schedule as a result of their children's health problems or the lack of adequate child care, poor women are often fired from or have to leave their service-sector jobs or find that they simply cannot continue when some family emergency occurs. Families can lose their child care subsidy when a parent loses her job or when a child is absent from child care too often. Such parents are considered to be inefficient users of the subsidy. Among the families we interviewed, however, work was rarely a route to health coverage in any case, and the expenses associated with employer-provided health coverage, when it was available at all, were prohibitive. Even for employed women, Medicaid and SCHIP were often the only coverage options for the family (although SCHIP was only recruiting families in Texas during our data-collection period), and so the families we spoke with had little experience with it.

Fragmented Family Coverage

Neither Medicaid nor any of the other publicly funded health insurance programs available to the poor provide family coverage. Rather, each member of the family falls into a different eligibility category depending on his or her age and the family's income. As a result of federal mandates, infants and young children are eligible in families with incomes even somewhat above the poverty threshold, but older children in the same family are often ineligible, and working-age adults, except for pregnant women and the seriously ill or disabled, do not qualify at all under the federal/state program (Davidoff et al. 2004). The result is that at any moment some family members might be enrolled in Medicaid or SCHIP whereas others might be covered by employer-based insurance and still others have no coverage. Such an incomplete and inconsistent system almost guarantees that there will be periods during which someone in the family will have no health insurance and needed care may have to be postponed. The only real alternatives are charity or the burdensome debt that medical expenditures impose on families with little discretionary income.

Tables 3.1 and 3.2 present data from the Three City Study survey that show the extent of incomplete individual and household health care coverage among poor families. In the first wave of the survey, we selected one "focal" child in each household for whom we collected detailed information, including information on his or her health care

TABLE 3.1. *Focal Child's and Caregiver's Insurance Status by City, Wave 1*

	Boston		Chicago		San Antonio	
Insurance Status	Focal Child	Caregiver	Focal Child	Caregiver	Focal Child	Caregiver
Employer or Union	12%	17%	15%	21%	15%	20%
Private/Military/Other	3%	5%	3%	2%	7%	10%
Medicaid	78%	74%	73%	69%	53%	48%
No Insurance	7%	4%	10%	8%	26%	21%

Note: Columns may not add up to 100% because of rounding.

TABLE 3.2. *Percentage of Households in Which All Children Are Covered by Caregiver's Insurance Status*

	All Children in the Household Insured		
Caregiver Insured	No	Yes	Total
No	89%	11%	100%
Yes	31%	69%	100%

coverage. We also collected information on health insurance sources for his or her caregiver, who in almost every case was the focal child's mother. In the second wave, we obtained detailed information on the health insurance coverage for each member of the family. Table 3.1 presents information from the first wave on the health insurance coverage of the focal child and his or her caregiver. It shows that in none of the three cities were a large percentage of focal children or their parents covered by employer-based or private health plans. For these families, Medicaid was the major source of coverage. Table 3.1 shows the substantial city differences in the rate of Medicaid coverage that will come up throughout our presentation. Medicaid coverage was substantially lower in San Antonio, both for the focal child and the mother, than in either Boston or Chicago. A far higher percentage of the San Antonio sample had no health insurance of any sort. These differences reflect state differences in eligibility criteria and other aspects of the program, as well as racial and ethnic differences that we will discuss in more detail throughout the book but especially in Chapter 6.

In Table 3.2, we present information from the second wave of the survey, in which we asked about the insurance status of every person in the household. In this table, we present the distribution of households in terms of whether the caregiver and all of the children in the household were covered by some form of health insurance. The first row of the table shows that in 89 percent of households in which the caregiver was not insured at least one child was also uninsured. Because the sample includes families with only one child, this statistic understates the problem. The probability of an uninsured child increases with the number of children in the family. The second row of Table 3.2 shows that even in households in which the caregiver had insurance 31 percent included one or more children who had no coverage and were not participating in Medicaid. As we will find throughout the following chapters, a parent's access to health insurance does not guarantee family coverage. As we noted in the discussion of our ethnographic interviews, the information provided by the respondents in our survey is probably not completely accurate because many mothers were unsure of or simply wrong about the actual enrollment status of every member of the family. Nonetheless, the patterns are probably generally correct, and we can be fairly certain that in a large fraction of low-income families, especially those with several children, some of the children have no health coverage.

Although the uninsured population no doubt includes some families who choose not to purchase available coverage that they might be able to afford, in this sample, as for low-income families in general, the lack of insurance is primarily involuntary and the result of structural problems related to the nature of employment-based health insurance coverage. As a consequence, many of the proposals for market-based health care financing reform, such as employer subsidies or medical savings accounts, that have been offered since the rejection of the Clinton plan are simply irrelevant for this population. Given the low earnings of the working poor, saving is nearly impossible, and even if a low-wage head of household is offered employer-based coverage, the probability that he or she would be able to afford full family coverage is low. Even when low-wage workers manage to obtain basic employer-sponsored coverage, the risk of losing that coverage is high (Williams et al. 2004). For employers, the increasing cost of health insurance means that a growing number do not offer coverage to their employees or they are requiring that workers shoulder an ever larger share of the cost (Blumberg and Holahan 2004a; Blumberg and Holahan 2004b; Hadley 2004; Lesser and Ginsburg 2003; Long and Shen 2004). As a result, more working Americans are simply priced out of the employer-based health insurance market. For adults and older children in uninsured low-wage families, there are almost no options for obtaining health care other than emergency rooms, charity, or crushing medical debt.

In this chapter, we begin our detailed journey into the health care experiences of low-income families and explore the strategies they employ to obtain and maintain health care coverage for at least some members of the family. We begin our examination by reviewing the causes and consequences of the episodic nature of health coverage for families who are dependent on public sources for care. The problems they encounter include difficulties in the application and recertification process for Medicaid, the often daunting nature of interactions with the welfare and health care systems, and the serious lack of coverage for adults. We tell the stories of families who struggled to make ends meet and to provide a decent life and health care for their children. We also present the stories of parents who, facing the realities of a system that does not provide health care to adults, do what they can for their children while giving up on getting care for themselves. We hear from parents who must make difficult choices about which of their children's health problems will get priority. Our presentation draws upon quantitative survey data as well, but the real story comes from the in-depth ethnographic interviews with families that were struggling to make ends meet.

These stories and the plight of many low-income families are wrenching, but these families are not simply victims. Many of them bring considerable strength and energy to their struggles, and some achieve real successes in overcoming serious obstacles. Yet after years of conducting research with the poor during which we have investigated the correlates of their access to health care, we knew that we would have to focus on the barriers that are a fundamental part of our system of health care financing and delivery. The stories we heard revealed many such barriers, as well as ongoing attempts to overcome them. In our interviews, health problems and the difficulties that poor parents faced in obtaining high-quality health care for their children and themselves came up often, even when the interview was focused on some other topic. Over and over we heard accounts of frequent and serious health problems, difficulties in "working" the public health care system, and sporadic employer-sponsored health care coverage that was available for a while when someone had a job but disappeared when a parent lost that job or could not afford to pay the premiums.

We heard numerous accounts of difficulties in obtaining Medicaid and of considerable delays in getting treatment for children's serious health problems. Because we were recruiting families into the study before SCHIP was implemented in Texas, the mothers of children who were ineligible for Medicaid had no choice but to rely on charity, go into debt, or do without medical care for uncovered children. The State Children's Health Insurance Program addressed a clear shortcoming in the system and increased the number of covered children considerably. The need it addresses is so great that even under the severe budgetary pressures faced by state legislatures following the 2000 economic downturn, it has enjoyed substantial public support (Hoadley, Cunningham, and McHugh 2004). Yet despite the clear need and the popularity of the program, financial problems have resulted in the curtailment of its expansion, and in some states, including Maryland, New York, and Texas, actual reductions in enrollment have occurred (Bergman, Williams, and Pernice 2004; Dunkelberg and O'Malley 2004; Smith, Rousseau, and O'Malley 2004).

In our interviews, we heard particularly harrowing accounts of parents doing without care for their own serious health problems. Although our system of health care financing takes pity on children, it shows little concern for the health care needs of their parents. Many parents struggled with health problems that prevented them from working and in some cases limited their ability to take care of their children. Some mothers we spoke with delayed routine health care for their children as well as for themselves when faced with choices between the risk of losing a job because of excess absences or taking their children to scheduled appointments. Because of the way the system works, we encountered situations in which parents were forced to pursue health care for one family member at a time while the needs of other family members had to be put on hold. What we brought away from these interviews was evidence of a seriously incomplete health care safety net that places children at serious risk of the long-term consequences of health problems, and that makes it very difficult for parents to maintain employment and achieve the self-sufficiency that is the stated objective of welfare reform.

TABLE 3.3. *Percentage of Focal Children and Caregivers without Coverage at Some Time in the Year Prior to the Initial Survey by City*

	City		
	Boston	Chicago	San Antonio
Focal Child	6%	8%	16%
Caregiver	8%	14%	17%

The Struggle to Maintain Coverage

As part of the first wave of the survey, we asked respondents whether there had been any period during the twelve months preceding the interview during which either they or the focal child had been without health care coverage. Unfortunately, the question included much missing data, revealing the difficulty that respondents have in answering retrospective questions about health care coverage. As the ethnographic data show, the volatility in coverage and the frequent confusion among parents regarding their children's coverage introduce errors into the data. Nonetheless, Table 3.3 reveals patterns that emerge throughout our analysis that largely reflect differences in state Medicaid policies. Whereas only 6 percent of focal children experienced some period without any coverage in Boston and 8 percent were without coverage at some time in Chicago, 16 percent of focal children were without coverage at some point during the previous year in San Antonio. Again these numbers are at times lower than those for the answer to the question as to whether the caregiver and the focal child were currently covered, but because of the missing data, the reference group is different. Nonetheless, even with errors, the pattern reveals the problem that we are facing. Among caregivers, periods of a lack of coverage were common and again reveal substantial differences among states. As we discuss in the next chapter, a higher fraction of caregivers in San Antonio are employed in jobs that do not offer any form of coverage than in either Boston or Chicago.

Another illustration of the lack of continuity of coverage is presented in Table 3.4, which shows the change in the focal child's Medicaid coverage during the year between the first and second interviews in each of the three cities. The ethnographic data made it clear that, given the volatility of Medicaid coverage, especially for older children, these figures on net change do not tell the whole story. During the course of

TABLE 3.4. *Change in Focal Child's Medicaid Status from Wave 1 to Wave 2*

	Boston	Chicago	San Antonio
Gain Medicaid	6%	9%	9%
Medicaid to Other Coverage	15%	17%	16%
Medicaid to Uninsured	4%	4%	13%
Kept Medicaid	75%	70%	62%

a year, eligibility can change more than once because recertification is required on a more frequent basis. The percentages in Table 3.4 show that over a relatively short period only 75 percent of children maintained their Medicaid coverage, even in Boston. In San Antonio, only 62 percent of children retained their Medicaid. The serious problem of uninsured children in Texas is revealed by the fact that 13 percent of the children who lost their Medicaid in San Antonio remained uninsured. As we noted earlier, we were personally responsible for the San Antonio ethnography and got to know the families who participated intimately. Because Texas leads the nation in the number of adults and children with no health care coverage of any sort, the city provides a unique view into the problems that poor families face in obtaining and maintaining coverage. In many ways, the state serves as an example of the logic of the more limited health care approach embodied in the new national desire to limit the government's role in welfare generally. In all three cities, enrolling a child in Medicaid was not simple; nor did initial success guarantee ongoing coverage. Only some of the families we interviewed in San Antonio were able to maintain health insurance coverage for all children continuously. As Table 3.5 shows, of the forty-five families in the ethnography whose health insurance we could track with certainty over time, only twenty-three were able to keep all of their children continuously covered, and only three of the women themselves had continuous coverage. Of those three women, only one was continuously covered by an employer-sponsored plan.

As we noted in our introduction to the ethnographic data, the complexity of the application and recertification procedures and the consequent lapses in coverage of which even the caregiver was unaware mean that these numbers are only approximate. Nonetheless, they clearly illustrate the fact that coverage was episodic. These figures are more

TABLE 3.5. *Discontinuities in Health Insurance: Mothers and Children*

	Mothers' Health Insurance Continuous	Mother's Health Insurance Discontinuous
Children's Health Insurance Continuous	3	23
Children's Health Insurance Discontinuous	0	19

Note: There are four cases for which information was sufficiently incomplete that coding into this chart was impossible.

dramatic than those from the survey for several reasons. First, we were able to double-check with families who believed they were covered to determine whether the individual whom the mother thought was covered was in fact insured. Second, families frequently experienced brief lapses in medical coverage because of difficulties in recertification. The mothers often did not tell us about these lapses or explain the reasons for them until we asked specifically about why they occurred and probed further. Third, families often counted access to low-cost medical care or to loans for medical purposes as health care insurance. Given the amount of time we spent with families in the ethnographic component, we were able to differentiate such instances from real health insurance. The ethnographic data therefore made it clear that survey researchers need to be conscious of the fact that the answers to simple questions concerning complex issues like health insurance coverage among low-wage families are plagued by potential errors that result from the uncertainty of poor people's insurance status or even their understanding of what constitutes health care coverage.

The strength of the ethnographic data, of course, is that they allowed us to observe the range of different strategies that mothers employed in order to obtain and maintain health insurance for their families. In order to illustrate just how different those strategies were, we present brief case studies of mothers' attempts to maintain coverage. As we will see, although some strategies were more successful than others, all had their shortcomings, and despite their best efforts most families experienced periods during which they lost coverage for at least one family member. Those resourceful families who were able to maintain continuous coverage were clearly in the minority. We present four cases, two of which were success stories in terms of maintaining family coverage and two of which reflect less successful strategies.

Darlene, an African American grandmother in her mid-forties, had primary responsibility for her two grandchildren, a growing trend among poor families in which parents lose custody of their children because they use drugs, are incarcerated, or for any number of other reasons are not up to the task of parenting. Darlene and her grandchildren relied on Medicaid, and she represents one of the rare cases in which a caregiver was able to make sure that she and her children were continuously eligible. Norma, a Latina mother of four, was also one of the success stories and one of the few mothers who was able to make use of employment-based coverage. Although she had experienced periods during which she and her children had no health insurance, she was able to maintain health coverage through her job almost continuously once she found employment. Leticia, another Latina mother in her twenties, had a much more difficult time maintaining coverage. She and her four sons moved between Medicaid coverage and periods with no health insurance. When Leticia and her children were without insurance, they were often forced to go without medical treatment. Anita, our final example, was a non-Hispanic white woman in her mid-thirties and described herself as a "white Puerto Rican." She was the mother of a three-year-old and also a teenager who did not live with her. The younger child, because of her age, was covered by Medicaid. Like many of the other women we interviewed, however, Anita herself had no insurance and was forced to go without treatment when she was ill or else had to pay for the care herself. The elaboration of each of these cases in more detail provides a window on the troublingly chaotic nature of health insurance from the perspective of a low-income family.

Darlene: Continuous Medicaid Coverage

Darlene was somewhat unusual among our families in being able to maintain almost continuous Medicaid coverage for herself as well as for the grandchildren in her care. The circumstances that led to Darlene's custody of her grandchildren reflect a fairly common contemporary reality and one that is difficult for everyone involved. Her situation was typical of that of a growing number of Medicaid-dependent households in which grandparents are forced to assume primary responsibility for their grandchildren. These grandparents must deal not only with the uncertainties related to their own health insurance coverage but also those related to their grandchildren's coverage. Darlene's daughter, the mother of the two children, lost custody of her older child at the time of the child's birth because she was using drugs and was determined by the courts to be an unfit parent. Although Darlene, who was in her mid-forties, was given custody of her granddaughter by the court, she was also raising her daughter's second child, a boy, even though she had not been granted custody of him. Darlene did not expect her daughter would ever assume direct responsibility for the children and was prepared to care for them until they grew up. Darlene depended on Medicaid for her grandchildren's medical care as well as her own, and she told us that she did not know how she could get care at all without it. As a consequence, the medical care she and her grandchildren received was determined entirely by what Medicaid would cover. As was the case for most of the caregivers in our sample, Darlene's efforts to maintain health insurance took place in the context of struggles to maintain a number of other services for herself and her grandchildren.

We first contacted Darlene in September 1999, when she lived in "Section 8" subsidized housing, a housing program for the poor that places poor families in privately owned apartments rather than in public housing. During the time we were in contact with her, she moved from housing that had been shut down to a new apartment with larger rooms. Although the cost of the move was considerable, Darlene greatly preferred the new apartment. Shortly after we met her, and following a considerable struggle, she qualified for supplemental security income (SSI), the program for disabled individuals that provides a more stable source of income, as well as medical coverage, than TANF or Medicaid. Individuals who qualify for SSI are not required to reestablish their eligibility for Medicaid as often as those who are not disabled. Darlene qualified for the program because of her poor health. She suffered from a range of health problems, including high blood pressure, chronic back and knee pain, hepatitis C, stomach pains, and depression and anxiety.

Darlene had five children of her own and a total of eight grandchildren, including the two who lived with her. In addition to caring for those two, she provided child care for as many as six of her grandchildren during the day while their parents worked. Because of what she described as her own failures as a parent, Darlene was very committed to providing this care for her grandchildren: As she said, "All they [her own children] saw was their mama on drugs, getting welfare, not working their whole life. If they can get up and go to work God will give me the strength to get up and take care of my grandchildren."

At the time of the first interview, before Darlene succeeded in her application for SSI, she and the two grandchildren who were living with her were on TANF. However, because of the then-new time limits, they had little more than one year of TANF eligibility left. Darlene was convinced that her poor health would prevent her from holding down a job, and her situation was increasingly desperate. Through it all, she continued with her long-term efforts to qualify for SSI. She and her two children also received Medicaid during this period, and although she worked at many jobs, she never had a job with benefits. She told us that she was once fired from a job just before the four-month probationary period required to receive benefits. For Darlene, the Medicaid for which she qualified as a TANF recipient before she qualified for SSI was critical because it allowed her to get care for her numerous medical conditions and to remain healthy enough to care for her grandchildren.

As important and valuable as Medicaid was to Darlene and the other families we interviewed, they expressed frustration with the problems they encountered in the process of qualification, recertification, and actually getting medical care even when they finally had Medicaid. Darlene, for example, reported that "When you go now [to the welfare office], you have some workers that act like that money comes out of their pockets. I have had some treat me like I wasn't human. They talk down to you. I still get nervous and kind of sick in the stomach when I go back for my six-month review because they do you so bad."

In November 1999, Darlene had to have some tests performed to diagnose the cause of chronic stomach pains. These tests revealed problems with her gallbladder that required surgery. After the surgery, she continued to experience pain and was referred to another doctor, who ordered more tests. However, when Darlene discovered that Medicaid would not pay for the tests, she decided not to have them. Darlene explained to us that there was a particular doctor she liked because she feels that he pays attention to her needs. She was told by Medicaid officials, however, that she had been to this doctor too often and that if her high use continued she would be placed in a special program to monitor her use of medical care. Darlene also explained that she had not been to a dentist for regular care in fifteen years because she did not receive dental benefits through Medicaid. When she had dental problems she could not ignore, she traveled across the city to the medical center at the university, where low-income people could get dental care for free.

In October 2000, Darlene was certified for SSI, just as she was about to reach her time limits on TANF. Although she appreciated the increase and stability in income that SSI provided, she experienced a new round of difficulties with her Medicaid. Prior to qualifying for SSI, one of Darlene's children had helped her enroll in a Medicaid managed-care plan that provided unlimited prescription drug coverage. This prescription coverage was critical because Darlene took seven different medications for her various health problems. However, when she switched to SSI, she was transferred to a form of Medicaid that only covered three prescriptions per month. Darlene's family practitioner helped her to deal with this limitation by prescribing each of her medications for three months at a time so she would not have to refill each one every month. That way, she was able to fill only three prescriptions in any given month. Unfortunately, the new plan did not pay for her psychiatric medications, which cost over $100 per prescription. Understanding and dealing with the exigencies of the different medical programs occupied much of Darlene's time during the period we were in contact with her.

Despite the limitations of Medicaid, private insurance was simply not an option for Darlene or her family. In discussing one of her children, who had one child and another on the way, she said, "Health insurance costs too much. On my daughter's job, she can only afford it for her; she can't afford it for her little girl. She's having a baby and can't afford it." Many of our families reported continued dependence on Medicaid, at least for their children, even when they were employed. Most employers in the low-wage job market they worked in did not offer health insurance and, in those cases in which it was offered, the employee contribution combined with co-pays and deductibles for medical services was unaffordable. By moving onto SSI, Darlene, unlike most adults, was able to continue her Medicaid coverage, and the children she cared for stayed eligible as well.

Norma: Continuous Coverage through Work

Norma was also unusual among the families we studied in her ability to acquire employer-assisted health insurance for her entire family. However, even though she managed to keep her health insurance during the time she was part of the study, she was continuously worried that she might lose the job that provided her family's health care coverage. The small bit of middle-class security she had managed to find was precarious. We contacted Norma for the first time in June 1999. At that time, she was a single mother with four children that ranged in age from one to eight. Norma had her first child when she was fifteen, and she had never finished high school. She and her children were living in public housing at the time of the first interview. Norma first began receiving welfare (then Aid to Families with Dependent Children, or AFDC) in 1991 after the birth of her first child. She received public assistance for between five and six years and left the rolls when her new husband, Pete, took over support of the family. Norma and Pete, the father of the two youngest children, were together for about four years, during which time the family did not receive welfare. Norma eventually left Pete because of his drinking.

At the time that we recruited her into the study, Norma was unmarried and had Medicaid for the children but not for herself. To obtain medical care for herself, she used a local hospital-based program that required payment based on a sliding payment scale for poor families that allowed them to make income-adjusted payments on their medical debt. The program also provided a partial subsidy for those who qualified, but only to the extent that the program's limited resources would allow. If participants make payments in accordance with a formula that determines how much they can afford to pay, they remain in good standing with the program and the participating medical facilities will continue to serve them. Such a situation, of course, can often result in the accumulation of debt because medical charges can build up far faster than a poor family can pay them.

Because of the inevitable debt she would incur, Norma avoided using medical services, occasionally going without care for serious medical problems. In the spring of 1999, for example, she had a serious rash that she left untreated. Although she saw a private doctor who charged her $50 to treat the problem, the cream he prescribed cost $65, an amount Norma could not afford to pay. As an alternative, she used a cream that her former mother-in-law had brought back from Mexico.

In 1999, Norma began a new job working on an assembly line. The employer offered a family health plan that included an employee premium. Norma debated about whether she should enroll the family in the plan or stay with the subsidized payment program. Finally, in June 2000, she decided to enroll the family in the plan, for which she paid a $40 monthly premium, a $10 co-payment for each doctor visit, a $50 co-payment for each emergency-room visit, and the full cost of prescription medications. Norma preferred employer-assisted insurance over Medicaid because of the public program's burdensome application process for each individual in the household. As she told us, "Over here with Medicaid you don't pay nothing, but you have to... prove everything, you have to go and be there for an hour till they help you or proved your Medicaid and all that." Although the insurance provided by her employer was costly, Norma preferred it, and she was just able to afford it given the relatively generous employer participation. However, like all employer-sponsored coverage, it is only as stable as the job. Manufacturing jobs are leaving San Antonio as they are many other American cities, and Norma remained concerned that if she lost her job she would lose not only income but the health coverage that came with it. Despite her worries, when we ended our interviews with Norma at the end of the research project, she was still employed and covered by her employer's plan.

Leticia: Times with No Medical Insurance, No Treatment – On and Off Medicaid

Leticia, who was not eligible for TANF, had no health insurance coverage herself, whereas her children were sometimes covered and at other times were not. Leticia joined the study in December 1999. She had four children, she had never finished high school, and she got her first job, at a fast food restaurant, just about the time we met her. At the time, she was receiving TANF for her two older children, whose father was in jail, and child support from the father of her two younger children. The family lived in public housing as part of a family self-sufficiency program. Leticia was not receiving TANF herself, nor was she on Medicaid. She was, in welfare terminology, a "child only" case. She told us that "They had me off of it [TANF] because when I got with my little ones' father, they told me I couldn't be on it because if I had a kid [child support] from him, he could support the other ones. That's what they told me."

In February 2000, one of her sons contracted ringworm but Leticia could not take him to the doctor because although she had reapplied for Medicaid she had not yet qualified. Her solution was to borrow some leftover medicine from her sister to treat the ringworm. As long as the child had the medical condition, Leticia's day care center would not allow him to attend because the condition is highly contagious. Leticia was unable to find another child care arrangement quickly enough to maintain her attendance at her GED classes, so she was dropped from the program.

In March 2000, Leiticia's eight-year-old son broke his arm, but he was not covered by Medicaid and Leticia was charged for his treatment. Luckily, that situation was resolved favorably and the child's Medicaid was restored. In one of our last interviews, she told us "I got my Medicaid now [for her son], so I called and gave them my Medicaid number." When we last saw Leticia, she was hoping that Medicaid would make retroactive payments for the expenses connected with her son's broken arm. We do not know whether she was successful in her attempt to get those costs covered.

Leticia, like many of the other families with whom we dealt, made decisions about medical treatment on the basis of whether the care was likely to be covered by Medicaid. Her inability to keep her children covered or to obtain complete and adequate medical treatment for them when they needed it had serious implications not only for the children's health but also for her employment and educational success. As in the case of so many of the other families, the lack of readily available medical care for her children meant that Leticia's attempts to further her own education and her capacity to hold a job were undermined by the absences required in order to deal with her children's health problems.

Anita: Going into Debt

Anita, even though she occasionally had health care coverage, had no choice but to go into debt to get the medical care she needed. Our first interview with her took place in July 1999. At the time, she was a thirty-five-year-old single parent who was living in public housing with her only child, a three-year-old daughter. Anita had a GED, and between the ages of nineteen and twenty-five she had held a number of low-paying jobs that included working as a waitress, a cook, and a convenience store clerk. Unfortunately, diabetes, back problems, and a degenerative knee disorder made continuing in those sorts of jobs impossible because they required that she be on her feet for most of the day and it was too painful and exhausting for her to do so. Health problems also interfered with Anita's educational ambitions. She had participated in Job Corps, a job preparation program, on two different occasions and had studied data processing at a junior college in south Texas during the 1992–93 academic year. However, she had been unable to complete the program because of a ruptured appendix. Anita's last job prior to our first interview was in 1996 driving people to work for a temporary employment service, a job that did not provide health insurance.

At the time of the first interview, Anita was enrolled in an intensive job-training and placement program. She graduated from that program in May 2001 with certification in "computers." It was unclear exactly what skills she had learned, however, and it also was not clear what kind of health insurance Anita had throughout this period. During the time we conducted our interviews with her, she was receiving TANF, and she had been on Medicaid since the birth of her child with only brief interruptions.

Although Anita welcomed the services she could get, TANF, she told us, is "a pain in the ass, literally. ... One thing about the Texas Department of Human Services, they do not volunteer information." Recounting one particularly exasperating encounter, Anita told of an occasion when she took her daughter for a well-child physical examination and shots during the same week that the girl turned four. At the clinic, she was told that she should have had the physical the month *after* the child turned four, although they did give the child her exam. In addition to Medicaid, the child was also covered by her father's insurance. Several families explained that the insurance provided by a nonresident father did not match the benefits of Medicaid and that as a consequence some children were allowed to remain on Medicaid. Despite the fact that the child had Medicaid and was on her father's insurance, Anita told us that she was still receiving medical bills. As she explained, "My Medicaid will cover what his insurance doesn't.

They're supposed to bill it to Medicaid, but I'm getting the bills ... it just piles up."

In 2001, as we conducted our final interviews with her, Anita was struggling to pay the medical costs she incurred as the result of her diabetes. Her medical debt was growing because of the chronic nature of the disease and the ongoing medical expenses she incurred. She explained that "If I need my [prescription] medicines, my Medicaid pays." But, like many mothers, she also faced expenses for over-the-counter supplies and medications that were not covered by Medicaid. "For my test strips and all that I have to go to the local hospital [hospital-based medical support program]." For other supplies, for food and body care, for eye care, and for other associated needs, she had to pay out-of-pocket. "But Medicaid says they have a program where they can pay for my test strips," she continued. Unfortunately, Anita did not have any more information about this program and was still paying for her test strips herself. She did not have dental coverage under Medicaid and received dental care through a university health system and the local hospital system. Because of her diabetes, her eye care was covered by Medicaid. Given the complexity of her chronic condition, however, Anita's debt was inevitably increasing. She knew that should she become employed or receive other income, she would be expected to repay the debt at a faster rate and very likely would lose her Medicaid coverage. For Anita and many others in our study, medical debt of this sort became a burden that they would never realistically pay off. Again, for these families, employment could easily make matters worse if it resulted in the loss of their Medicaid.

Health Care Coverage for the Poor: Few Choices

These cases reveal serious shortcomings in the health care safety net for poor families and illustrate the pervasiveness and seriousness of the health problems from which they suffer. Historically, the poor have found themselves at significantly elevated risk of both chronic health conditions and the more acute problems that stem from infectious disease, accidents, and violence (Institute of Medicine 2001; Link and Phelan 1995; Williams and Collins 1995; Winkleby and Cubbins 2003). This means that the poor experience a double jeopardy that results from the fact that they have the most serious and complex medical care needs at the same time that they are the least likely to have continuous access to adequate medical services (Institute of Medicine 2002a). They are confronted with the daily reality of having to choose among food, housing, or health insurance (Long 2003). Our interviews clearly showed that the struggle to maintain even sporadic coverage for family members is time consuming, difficult, and very likely to create problems in other areas of life. As we saw, poor health can interfere with the ability of a parent to hold down a job, and the health problems of anyone in the family can undermine the educational potential and aspirations of both children and adults.

Our interviews also showed that parents in low-wage jobs face a serious dilemma in reconciling work and the need to get medical care for their children. When their children are ill and need medical attention, at the very least they lose badly needed income. Some, however, face the very real risk of losing their jobs because of excessive absences. For parents with children who suffer from chronic health problems such as asthma, the situation is even more serious because of the ongoing nature of their child's health care needs. For many of the families in our study, the accumulation of health problems and the difficulties they created undermined parents' attempts to stay steadily employed and to save any money at all. After spending time with these families, we came to realize that the lack of full family coverage is a major structural problem in the United States.

A number of families with young children lacked medical coverage for at least some children for substantial periods (Cunningham and Park 2001), and an even larger number experienced fluctuations in medical coverage that were difficult to understand and manage. The time and effort required to maintain coverage and to requalify after a child has been dropped from Medicaid could easily undermine a parent's ability to act as a responsible employee. Even a middle-class family with economic resources and some job flexibility faces serious challenges in meeting the health care needs of a child with a chronic condition. For parents in low-wage work, such flexibility rarely exists. In addition, many of the parents in impoverished families are too ill themselves to succeed in the workforce. A large number of studies show that the adults in families that leave the TANF rolls who do not enter the labor force are very often in poor health (Loprest 2003a; Moffitt 2002; Moffitt and Winder 2003). Many cannot work because they are not healthy enough to do so.

As the literature we cited shows, the longer a family is off welfare the more likely it is that someone in the household will lose his or her health insurance. Such a situation penalizes work and the attempts that families make to become self-sufficient. Given that self-sufficiency is the core objective of welfare reform, such a situation is illogical and contradictory. The data also tell an important story concerning the role of race and ethnicity in defining the risk of inadequate health care coverage. The educational and occupational disadvantages that minority Americans suffer are compounded by a lack of adequate health care coverage. Minority Americans therefore face a triple jeopardy in terms of health care. The fact that minority Americans find themselves at particularly high risk of poor health with no health care coverage is no accident (Quadagno 1994). Our data revealed particularly serious problems for Mexican Americans. The disadvantages that they face in the labor force almost guarantee compromised health and inadequate coverage. Mexican Americans are the most severely underinsured population in the nation (Berk, Alberts, and Schur 1996; Doty and Ives 2002; Giachello 1992; Halfon et al. 1997; Iannotta 2002; Lillie-Blanton, Leigh, and Alfaro-Correa 1996; Santos and Seitz 2000; Valdez et al. 1993; Zambrana and Logie 2000). As we show in greater detail in Chapter 6, the combination of disadvantages that they face place these families at particularly high risk of poor health and inadequate coverage.

The Illogic of Welfare: The Marriage Penalty

One can hardly spend much time with poor families without arriving at the realization that many aspects of current welfare policy contradict its intended objective of encouraging at least some degree of self-sufficiency and marital stability. One such illogical policy consequence relates to the marriage penalty for Medicaid. Families that are receiving cash assistance or those that are in or near poverty qualify for Medicaid and other social welfare services. These families consist disproportionately of single mothers with dependent children. Meanwhile, two-parent households in which one or both adults are employed in

TABLE 3.6. *Percentage of Households
in Which All Children Have Health
Insurance by Mother's Marital Status*

Cohabiting	69%
Separated	71%
Single	71%
Married, Spouse Present	60%

low-wage jobs are the least likely to have medical insurance. Table 3.6 presents data from the second wave of the Three City Survey in which we collected health care information for all children in the household. It shows the percentage of households in which all children are covered by the marital status of the mother and clearly reveals the penalty associated with marriage.

Compared with households in which a single mother is the head, households that include the mother's partner are less likely to have complete health care coverage for all children. Multivariate analyses that are presented elsewhere show that even after controlling for household income, the education of the mother, race and ethnicity, and more, the penalty remains and cannot be attributed to higher incomes among two-parent households (Angel, Frias, and Hill 2005). Unfortunately, the presence of a male can raise income just enough to move the household just high enough to make at least the older children ineligible for public programs even when the parents' jobs do not provide employer-sponsored coverage or enough of a salary to purchase private insurance. If one of the intended objectives of welfare policy is to encourage marriage, a situation in which marriage reduces the likelihood of family medical care coverage is a clear marriage penalty.

We found that the loss of health care coverage is only one of the potential penalties that marriage brings. Marriage can result in the loss of many other essential benefits. Because they have higher marriage rates, Mexican Americans are particularly vulnerable to the marriage penalty. Mexican Americans face numerous structural disadvantages. They are at high risk of unemployment and poverty at the same time that they find themselves penalized by the unintended consequences of policies that supposedly encourage marriage and responsible parenthood when in fact they often do the opposite. The data clearly show that individual and group-specific vulnerabilities interact with state policies and local labor markets to place certain Americans at elevated risk of poor health and the lack of full access to health care.

We found other illogical aspects of the support system for low-wage individuals and families that clearly penalize marriage and work. The fact that a family is at risk of losing its health insurance when a parent becomes employed, even in a job that does not offer benefits, is hardly an incentive to work. In the United States, the combination of employer-based health care and public health insurance for some groups of poor people and the elderly leaves a large fraction of the population uncovered and handicapped in their capacity for economic and social mobility. Although the lack of continuous health insurance is certainly not the only difficulty faced by low-income families in the United States, it is a central problem that affects employment, access to child care, children's school attendance, and a host of other measures of family well-being. Low-income families, particularly those that have never been on welfare or that have received it sporadically, as well as those families headed by a married couple, face all of the risks associated with irregular health insurance.

As serious as the problem of the total lack of health care coverage in the United States may be, we also face a serious problem associated with underinsurance, a term we use to characterize the incomplete and episodic coverage we have described in this chapter. The phenomenon of underinsurance affects far more than the nearly fifty million Americans who have no insurance at all at any moment. The uncertainty that incomplete coverage introduces into family life and the health risks it entails undermine health and the ability of struggling families to get ahead. For a middle-class family, enrolling in an employer's health plan occurs when or shortly after one is initially hired, during an annual enrollment period, or when one acquires a new dependent. For unemployed and working poor families, the struggle to maintain coverage is ongoing and, as our ethnographic interviews revealed, often means that someone in the family must do without needed medical care. Although the problems associated with health insurance vary somewhat from place to place, as we show in Chapter 4, even the more generous policies of some states leave families facing serious health insecurities.

4

State Differences in Health Care Policies and Coverage

San Antonio

San Antonio is a very "Mexican" city. Over half of its population is Hispanic, 70 percent of whom are of Mexican origin (Guzmán 2001). Like many other cities in the American Southwest, it sprawls over an immense area, and even in the barrio the presence of many undeveloped areas gives it a feeling of openness. In latitude, the city is North African, and the days are long even in winter. The climate is temperate to hot, and when the rare snow falls, children younger than five or six are usually seeing it for the first time. The city's tourism industry, which is an important source of its income, capitalizes upon its visible Mexican heritage. The city's Mexican heritage can be seen in popular tourist sites such as the Alamo, cultural museums, native marketplaces, and theme parks that focus on Texas history.

Until Texas claimed its independence in the early nineteenth century, it was part of Mexico. The Alamo, an old Spanish mission that occupies a prominent place in the center of town, is known to all Americans as a legend that serves as the shrine of Texas liberty for the Anglo population. For many Mexican-origin Americans, however, it represents something quite different. For them the Mexican victory at the Alamo was short-lived and represents the beginning of an ultimate defeat and the start of a period during which the Mexican population was relegated to the rank of second-class citizens. The vast majority of the Mexican-origin population of the United States, of course, cherishes its U.S. citizenship, and those who are not citizens struggle to become Americans. Mexican Americans, and even Mexican nationals, have fought in all of America's wars, and many have moved into the economic and social mainstream. Yet, like African Americans, the unique history of the Mexican-origin population in this country has not included full economic and social incorporation for the group as a whole. Many Mexican-origin individuals in the United States remain outsiders to at least some degree. Some, of course, arrived only recently, and others are undocumented immigrants who live among us just below the surface of everyday life. Their marginal status is not surprising. Yet even for many of those who have been Americans since Texas and the rest of the Southwest became part of the United States, full incorporation has not occurred. Mexican American education levels, incomes, and personal wealth remain far below those of the majority non-Hispanic white population (Angel and Angel 1997; Grogger and Trejo 2002; Suro 1998).

Downtown San Antonio is dominated by hotels, museums, tourist attractions, and office and municipal buildings. The municipal core is only a mile from one of the poorest neighborhoods in the city, in which we carried out part of our study. Unlike the Midwest, San Antonio's economy was never defined by large smokestack manufacturing. In the years after World War II, some small-scale manufacturing jobs were available, but most of those have disappeared. Plants ranging from a blue jeans factory to a meat packing plant have closed since the 1990s, leaving the city largely dependent on tourism, health care, and the service sector for its economic base. Military installations continue to represent an important part of the local economy.

As in Boston and Chicago, neighborhoods differ from one another even when they share a basically similar socioeconomic profile. One defining characteristic of many San Antonio neighborhoods is the presence of large low-rise public housing projects and other apartment-style low-income housing. Some of our study neighborhoods were defined by such projects, whereas others included more single-family houses and private apartments. A few of our San Antonio families lived in The Courts, a public housing project that covers close to three-quarters of a square mile less than a mile from downtown. The Courts, however, like most San Antonio developments, differed from the old high-rise apartment complexes that are typical of Chicago and Boston. San Antonio projects more often consist of street after street of one- or two-story buildings that contain small apartments. The Courts is one of the old-est housing projects in the south, originally dedicated in a ceremony attended by then First Lady Eleanor Roosevelt. During the hot San Antonio summer, doors and windows stand open because the apart-ments are not air-conditioned and indoor temperatures reach well over one hundred degrees. Many of the small yards in front of the housing units contain small flower gardens and wading pools that are among the few sources of beauty and recreation visible.

Most residents stay fairly close to home, except when they are forced to travel for work, to shop, or to obtain services. We met families whose school-age children had never been to the nearby downtown. Public transportation was inadequate and often involved a long walk to an inconveniently located bus stop. The city has no commuter train or subway system, and getting around the city is a constant problem for poor families. Although San Antonio is home to a major university health science center, its health care resources are concentrated on the outskirts or downtown and families using them must take long trips on public transportation. The only grocery store serving the same neighborhood is a small bodega, or what might be characterized as a mom and pop convenience store, although a supermarket opened roughly a mile away during the time of our study. At a somewhat greater distance, one could find a clinic that accepted Medicaid. To shop for major items or to obtain care for serious health problems, residents have to travel beyond the immediate neighborhood, which almost always represents a major effort. For the most part, only the most basic medical care is locally available, and our respondents used public transportation or found a ride to get to the doctor or clinic. Because most of our families did not own a car, their limited access to transportation also restricted the jobs they could take.

Chicago

Far to the northeast of San Antonio lies Chicago, in the agricultural and manufacturing heartland of the nation. As is the case in most American cities, in Chicago the movement of manufacturing jobs overseas means that the service sector accounts for a growing proportion of jobs, espe-cially for the poor and those who have recently arrived. More massive and older urban structures and a longer, gray winter give Chicago a very different feel than San Antonio. Chicago provides a real sense of the intensity of urban America. Although San Antonio is home to nearly half a million individuals who trace their lineage to Mexico, the fairly recent migration of Mexicans to the Midwest has given Chicago an even larger Mexican-origin population (Guzmán 2001; Suro and Singer 2002). The city's Mexican-origin population is second only to that of Los Angeles in size. The city also contains large Puerto Rican and African American populations.

Chicago has been likened to a mosaic because of the clear distinctions among its many neighborhoods. As immigrant groups arrived, they occupied particular parts of the city and gave each its unique identity, in addition to well-defined boundaries. Like the Poles, Croatians, Lithuanians, Italians, and other groups who in years past lived in the same neighborhoods, the relatively new Mexican arrivals have redefined Pilsen/Little Village, one of the neighborhoods where we worked, which stretches from the Chicago River on its eastern border to the city limits on its western edge, and from around 16th Street on its north side to the Stevenson Expressway on its southern edge. This area is clearly a Mexican domain but one that exists in a physical environment very different from that of the Southwest.

Today, Chicago has a complex economy that includes manufacturing and service jobs. It is also home to several medical schools with associated teaching hospitals and clinics. Nevertheless, like San Antonio, it does not have the rich assortment of neighborhood clinics and health services available in many Boston neighborhoods. Unlike San Antonio, however, the city has a highly developed and dependable public transportation system, and getting to services is relatively easy. Given the clear dominance of local neighborhoods, most of the residents of the neighborhoods we studied stayed close to home and ventured out of their local neighborhoods only for services that were not available close by. When they had to travel, they had access to relatively straightforward transportation that, unlike San Antonio, made the use of services easier.

Boston

Boston, one of the nation's oldest cities, has always been racially and ethnically diverse, but today it is taking on the new Latino flavor. The city has a growing Hispanic population that is primarily Puerto Rican and Dominican. It also has a large African American population. As in other cities, Hispanics and African Americans are concentrated in the poorer neighborhoods, such as Roxbury and Jamaica Plain. Although with Chicago and San Antonio it shares many of the characteristics of larger cities, including the racial/ethnic concentration of poverty in particular neighborhoods, it is unique in many important ways. Perhaps most notably, it has a greater diversity of jobs. Service-sector job growth has certainly outpaced that in any other sector, but the city and surrounding region also offer opportunities for employment in light manufacturing and the high-tech industry. Unfortunately, few of these opportunities were available to our study families.

The Boston area includes numerous colleges, universities, and technical education centers, and it was an early center for the high-tech industry. The city's economy also depends on an extensive tourism industry driven by the numerous historical sites related to the nation's colonial period. It is also a national health research and education center with numerous medical schools, hospitals, and specialty clinics. Despite adopting relatively stringent welfare reform regulations, Boston has historically embodied a progressive political tradition and a generous social welfare philosophy. The city offers the poor a wealth of health and child care options, educational programs, and other assistance programs at the local level. The city has an efficient and extensive public transportation system, and getting to services was relatively easy for the respondents in our study. Housing is very expensive in Boston, and poor families rely on government subsidies for housing to a larger extent than in Chicago or San Antonio.

Roxbury, a traditionally black community south of the downtown area, is made up of distinct neighborhoods that range from deeply impoverished areas to areas occupied by middle-class families. A walk down any street in a low-income neighborhood in Roxbury reveals a range of housing. One public housing project, "The Blues," in which we conducted some of our interviews, consists of a series of buildings four to eight stories high that are connected by paved walkways. Although Boston, like Chicago, is moving away from its earlier reliance on high-rise public housing, the newer housing still consists of a series of shorter towers with interior hallways and elevators that can be dark and frightening. In Boston, projects are categorized in terms of the neighborhood in which they are located and by whether they are the old-style high-rise or one of the newer townhouse designs. The taller buildings are part of the older public housing stock that is still in use. During the 1970s and 1980s, the massive high-rise projects a few miles away in Dorchester were transformed into mixed-use facilities. Despite all of the changes that have occurred in public housing and in Boston neighborhoods, those in which we conducted our interviews revealed a great stability. The mothers in our study grew up in or near the same neighborhoods in which they now live with their children.

The Blues offers its residents many local conveniences and services. The project is located about a block away from a commercial area that includes a number of shops, ranging from beauty salons and restaurants to music and clothing stores. Half a mile away, there is a more extensive business area with grocery stores, a number of different human services agency offices, and a health clinic. The intermediate area is quite varied and includes several blocks of large, renovated Victorian houses in a neighborhood that has been gentrified. As is the case for most Boston residents, public transportation is readily available. Within two and a half blocks of The Blues, a subway station connects the project with the rest of the city. The subway line that serves this neighborhood goes directly to the downtown area and then on to Cambridge and other out-lying areas. Although the subway system is built on a hub-and-spoke model and often requires transfers to complete a journey, the speed of the subway and the short connections reduce the travel time necessary to reach many services. The large teaching hospitals in Boston and their multiple clinics are easily reached by subway. Although Boston is also served by a bus system, the subway provides a speedy and often more useful alternative.

Three Different Political, Cultural, and Social Environments

As these portraits reveal, our three cities are very different in their physical and social environments. The state policies that govern their welfare programs are also about as different as possible. Massachusetts represents one extreme in the generosity of its welfare programs and Texas the other in the extent of limitations on eligibility and the extent of coverage of the population in need. Yet, as we explain in this chapter, we found through our ethnographic interviews that the realities of poverty and the challenges inherent in dealing with welfare bureaucracies largely overwhelmed these differences. Although families in San Antonio were considerably more likely than families in the two other cities to experience periods without health care coverage, in all three cities families shared many of the same frustrations and difficulties that seem to be an inevitable part of dealing with the means-tested public health care system, as well as other welfare bureaucracies. Regardless of where they lived, our families were remarkably similar in terms of their health levels and the irritations and frustrations they faced in obtaining and maintaining family health coverage. One San Antonio case was typical of stories we heard in all three cities.

Natalie

During one of our early interviews with her, Natalie, a Latina mother of three daughters who was in her thirties, described what it was like to go through the process of recertification for Medicaid. With considerable exasperation, she said "I've got to plan a whole day just to go and do this...because it takes so long!" One day she had an eight-thirty appointment to meet with her social worker to recertify her Medicaid eligibility. When she arrived at the office, she turned in the paperwork she was required to bring and sat down to wait with all of the other parents who also had eight-thirty appointments. After a long wait, someone came into the waiting room and called the names of those who were to be seen first, including Natalie. That group was ushered into a classroom where they were required to listen to a lecture on Medicaid that covered eligibility criteria and a range of other matters. After the presentation, each parent was called in to see the caseworker individually. As Natalie noted, "You're lucky if you're the first one called by your caseworker. If you're not, you have to wait until he goes through all the clients and gets to you." If you are one of the last called, you can wait all day, as Natalie had often done.

Depending on the nature of the administrative problem she was facing, Natalie was sometimes able to request what she called an "individual appointment" with her caseworker. When she managed to get such an appointment, she did not have to listen to the lecture on program rules before seeing her caseworker. Also, when she had a fixed appointment she felt more justified in complaining if she had to wait too long because she had to take time off from work, travel to the welfare office, and give up needed income. Of course, she explained, any complaint usually fell on deaf ears. Individual meetings with her caseworker, however, usually went routinely, and after processing the necessary paperwork Natalie could be on her way. Even short and efficient meetings, however, were disruptive and required time off from work. The recurring need to recertify each of her children separately was stressful and time consuming, and the effort was not always successful. The application and recertification procedures for the programs she used required that Natalie miss a lot of work and, as was the case for other mothers in our study, she had to placate her supervisor and on occasion she ran the risk of losing her job.

Natalie, in fact, did lose her job because of health problems, and then in a cruel bureaucratic irony almost simultaneously lost her own Medicaid at a time when she needed it most. The circumstances surrounding the job loss and the loss of her Medicaid were complex and began when she had to have a hysterectomy because of extensive bleeding that was the result of uterine tumors. On this occasion, the fact that Natalie was employed worked to her disadvantage. As part of the Medicaid recertification process, she had recently reported her income to the Medicaid office and lost her eligibility because with her slightly increased income she no longer met the means test. Unfortunately, just as she lost her Medicaid she was fired as the result of excessive health-related absences. The income-based payment plan we mentioned earlier was her only real alternative for paying for her health care, and she used it when she could. However, without insurance and without a job, she was forced to take out a loan to pay her medical bills. For poor families such as Natalie's, one problem often precipitates a number of other problems that culminate in a catastrophic outcome.

Like so many others in her situation, Natalie had a checkered work history, and none of her jobs provided health insurance either for herself or her children. Although her daughters were periodically on Medicaid, Natalie had coverage for herself only during her pregnancies. After graduating from high school, Natalie began working as a full-time cashier at a department store, but she left that job when she was accused of stealing. She took another job at a bowling alley, but once she had divorced her first husband, she could no longer support herself and her daughter on the salary that job paid. She then took a better-paying job at a pawn shop. In this new job, Natalie had to leave her youngest child with a friend because she had to work until 5:30 P.M., after which she had an hour commute. She could not find other child care that would allow her to pick the child up as late as 6:30 P.M. She lost the job at the pawn shop when she had her hysterectomy.

In light of the gravity of her health problems, and in order to help the family out while Natalie was jobless and ill, her partner, the father of her second child, moved in with her. This precipitated yet another crisis because the family was living in subsidized housing that did not allow another adult to move in, especially an adult male who in the eyes of the authorities should support the family. When the partner's presence was discovered, Natalie and her daughters were evicted and she had to move in with her mother. While she was living with her mother and recovering from the surgery, she tried to find work. She was particularly worried about paying back the large debt that she incurred as the result of her operation. Throughout this period, Natalie was also trying to help her grandmother, who had recently moved to San Antonio from Mexico City. The old woman, who had been ill, died toward the end of the time that we were in contact with Natalie, and the loss represented yet another negative event that added to the chaos of her family life.

Some months after these events, Natalie found a new job at a different pawn shop and slowly began to get back on her feet. Shortly afterward, however, she injured her back and knee during a particularly strenuous day of moving and lifting, and she was unable to get out of bed the next morning. Although her doctor prescribed therapy for the job-related injury, she was still without health insurance and her employer would not pay for the treatment. Nearly destitute and in need of treatment, Natalie managed to qualify for Medicaid for a twelve-month period. Despite almost constant back pain, she had to get to work and also get to her therapy appointments. Her mother tried to help, but Natalie worried that her mother might well lose her own job if she took too much time off from work to help out.

Natalie often experienced moments of discouragement and felt that she was only barely living up to her responsibilities. With so many crises in her life, she often felt little hope for the future. She could only dream about the impossible luxury of a vacation and a respite from all of the demands of her life. Fantasizing, she told us, "I'd like a hotel room somewhere for a week where I could take hot baths with candles and music to help me relax." But she continued with her daily routine, hiding her worries from her mother and children. She admitted that whatever semblance of normal feelings she displayed was just a front to hide her real desperation: "I keep my face strong, so nobody will know I am weak. It's a bluff."

Would It Be Different in Another City?

Natalie lived in Texas, a state with some of the weakest supports for poor families in the country and the one with the highest proportion of uninsured citizens in the nation. As we described, San Antonio provides only limited public transportation, and getting to health care and other services is difficult and time consuming. We have argued that Texas serves as the extreme example of the consequences of the limited programmatic support for poor families that are increasingly part of limited budgets and public hostility to welfare. This hostility resulted in competition among states to limit benefits, resulting in what some have described as a "race to the bottom" (Albert and Catlin 2002). Although poor families in San Antonio faced particularly serious problems related to transportation and very low welfare payments, families in Boston and Chicago were in reality no better off, especially because the cost of living is so much higher in those cities. The three cities in our study are all large metropolitan areas in states with very different welfare policies, and our objective was to determine how that variation might affect families' experiences with health care and health insurance. In addition to differences in welfare policies, the cities were chosen because they represent three important regions of the country, with unique labor markets, and unique mixes of metropolitan resources such as public transportation and housing, and unique health service environments. They also differ in their racial and ethnic compositions, a consideration very important to our objective.

San Antonio has a large and growing minority population and according to census figures is 58 percent Hispanic, and these Hispanics are primarily of Mexican origin (Guzmán 2001). Although nearly half a million individuals of Mexican origin live in San Antonio, Chicago's Mexican-origin population is larger as a result of increasing immigration since 1960. Boston has a large and growing Puerto Rican population, as does Chicago, but its Hispanic population also consists of Dominicans, Salvadorans, Mexicans, and other Central and South

Americans (Boston Redevelopment Authority 2001; Gusmán 2001). Chicago and Boston have larger African American populations than does San Antonio, although all three cities contain large numbers of African Americans, who reside mostly in minority neighborhoods, and like much of the rest of the United States, all three cities include growing Asian populations (U.S. Bureau of the Census 2000).

In this chapter, we compare the cities in terms of the completeness of health care coverage for poor families using data from the Three City Study survey, examine the broad social and economic environments of the three cities, and summarize differences in their eligibility rules for Medicaid and other health programs. We present data from the ethnography that illustrate the difficulties families face in maintaining continuous coverage in all three places. The ethnographic data reveal the ongoing struggle required to maintain health care coverage and the relative disadvantage of powerless individuals in dealing with complex, and what at times seem like arbitrary and hostile, bureaucracies. The differences that emerge among the three cities relate not only to their different welfare policies but also to geography, the local transportation and health care delivery systems, and the local labor market. Although state welfare policies, including those related to health care, differ in important ways, no matter where they lived, our families faced difficult challenges in maintaining public health coverage for the whole family even when they qualified for it initially. Once again, the data make it clear that the core problem arises from the lack of a universal health care system and the reliance on employer-based health insurance in the nation as a whole.

Boston families in the ethnographic sample had far fewer problems with continuity of health insurance than did San Antonio families. This seemed to be related primarily to the far greater generosity of MassHealth, the Massachusetts Medicaid program that covered children up to 200 percent of the federal poverty line (FPL) and their caretakers up to 133 percent of the FPL. In addition, in Boston, a somewhat larger number of families than in Chicago or San Antonio had access to some level of employer health care coverage. The causes of discontinuities in coverage also differed between Boston and San Antonio. In San Antonio, our families experienced periods of ineligibility because of more restrictive eligibility criteria as well as a lack of coverage when paperwork did not flow smoothly. Boston families experienced discontinuous health care coverage of shorter duration primarily when there was some difficulty with the paperwork. Chicago families' experiences fell somewhere between those of families in Boston or San Antonio.

Even in Boston, however, health care coverage for families was neither seamless nor administratively simple. Although the range of care covered was broader than in Texas, it had some important limitations. In all three cities, families lacked coverage for eye care and glasses, and they had only limited dental coverage. Although Massachusetts was unusual in providing treatment for at least some mental health conditions, no state provides public insurance coverage for all mental health conditions or all of the treatment they require. Because of Texas' historically restrictive welfare policies, even before welfare reform San Antonio embodied the new national mood that has changed the context of welfare and health care for low-income families. Texas and San Antonio moved toward more restrictive policies well in advance of the federal legislation through the use of waivers (Capps et al. 2001). As we have noted, in many ways Texas represents the logical culmination of the process of devolution in a time of restricted budgets. Without a state income tax and in the face of the post-2000 economic slowdown, the insurance situation for the poor in Texas deteriorated (Dunkelberg and O'Malley 2004; Smith, Rousseau, and O'Malley 2004). Although the retrenchment may have been more pronounced in Texas than in Massachusetts or Illinois, similar changes were introduced in those states as well, largely mandated by federal law but also reflecting state initiatives. All three cities therefore embodied the new opposition to cash assistance and time-limit preferences that spread across the nation in the 1990s. As a result of welfare reform, all three cities experienced a significant retrenchment in eligibility for welfare and other public benefits. At the same time, all three cities experienced declines in manufacturing employment and a growth in the proportion of low-wage service-sector jobs (Anari and Datzour 2004; Boushey and Rosnick 2004; Kalleberg, Reskin, and Hudson 2000).

The Drop in Medicaid Coverage after Welfare Reform

After the implementation of federal welfare reform in 1996, Illinois, Massachusetts, and Texas experienced dramatic drops in Medicaid enrollment, as did every other state (Chavkin, Romero, and Wise 2000; Committee on Child Health Financing 2001; Ku and Bruen 1999; Rowland, Salganicoff, and Keenan 1999). This decline occurred even as states increased spending on Medicaid and in spite of the fact that the majority of children who were not enrolled qualified on the basis of income (Holahan and Bruen 2003; Kohn, Hasty, and Henderson 2002; Rowland, Salganicoff, and Keenan 1999; Starfield 2000). This drop in Medicaid was a clearly unintended consequence of welfare reform, the objective of which was primarily to limit cash assistance. In response to the fact that many children in near-poor families do not qualify for Medicaid, Congress provided funding for the State Children's Health Insurance Program (SCHIP), which offers coverage to children not eligible for Medicaid because their family's income is too high. All three states now have an operating SCHIP program, although during the time of our study Texas was just beginning to enroll children.

Even after the introduction of SCHIP, however, many eligible children remain uninsured (Chavkin, Romero, and Wise 2000; Dubay, Haley, and Kenney 2002; Kohn, Hasty, and Henderson 2002; Ku and Bruen 1999; Salsberry 2003; Weinick and Krauss 2000; Zuckerman et al. 2001). Although Texas finally began enrolling children in SCHIP, the state has since dropped children from its SCHIP program because of serious state budgetary shortfalls. In 2003, the drop in Texas' SCHIP enrollment was in fact so dramatic that it resulted in a national decrease in the number of children covered (Dunkelberg and O'Malley 2004). As our ethnographic data reveal, even the rather dramatic statistics concerning the number of uninsured children in all three cities do not fully reveal the true extent of the problem of incomplete and inadequate health care coverage for either children or adults. As we reiterate throughout this book, families in all three cities faced the recurring problem of frequent, if relatively short, lapses in coverage because of bureaucratic roadblocks or errors.

State Medicaid Policies

In all states, in order for a child to qualify for Medicaid, his or her family had to fall below income thresholds that vary with the child's age (Health Care Financing Administration 2000). By 2003, states were required to cover all children under nineteen in families with incomes below 100 percent of the federal poverty line (FPL), although not all states had done so at the time of our study. At the time we were recruiting families, the federal government required states to cover children less than six years of age in families with incomes below 133 percent of the FPL. Even today, although the federal government sets the basic eligibility standards, the states retain a good deal of discretion in setting eligibility standards and payment levels within those federal mandates. As a consequence, the Medicaid eligibility requirements for children in Illinois, Massachusetts, and Texas differ significantly. As of July 2000, while we were carrying out our interviews, Illinois covered infants less than one year of age in families with income at or below 200 percent of the federal poverty line. In that state, children up to nineteen in families with incomes below 133 percent of the FPL were also covered. Massachusetts covered infants at or below 200 percent of the FPL, whereas older children nineteen and younger were covered at or below family incomes of 150 percent of the FPL.

Texas had far more restrictive eligibility policies than either Illinois or Massachusetts for older children (Capps 2001; Ross and Cox 2000). In Texas, infants below one year of age were eligible for Medicaid if they lived in families with incomes at or below 185 percent of the FPL. Children between the ages of one and five qualified only if their family's income fell below 133 percent of the FPL, and children between six and nineteen years of age were eligible only if their family income was below the federal poverty threshold. Caregivers were excluded from Medicaid unless they were receiving SSI, were disabled, or were pregnant (Health Care Financing Administration 2000; Strayhorn 2001). Texas formally covered the medically needy, but the income and asset limits required to qualify were extremely low. The state did not have a state-financed health coverage program for families that did not qualify for Medicaid. Rather, it relied on public hospitals run by the counties to provide indigent care. In 1997, the Texas Healthy Kids Corporation, a public/private partnership, began providing health insurance to nearly 1.3 million uninsured children ages two through eighteen. Although this program required that a family pay a monthly premium for each child covered, it also offered assistance through private funding in paying the premium for families with low incomes. During the 2001 legislative session, Texas passed legislation to simplify the application procedure for Medicaid.

In contrast with Texas, Massachusetts has attempted to cover as many poor families as possible, often at state expense. Under a federal waiver, the state greatly expanded its coverage of the poor through MassHealth. This program covered pregnant women and infants less than one year of age in families with incomes below 200 percent of the FPL and all children up to age nineteen in families with incomes below 150 percent of the FPL. The state's SCHIP program is part of MassHealth and was approved in 1998 with a retroactive start date of July 1997. Massachusetts also provides health care coverage to the poor and unemployed through several other state-funded insurance programs, including an uncompensated care pool that provides coverage for hospital care. As a result of its generous policies, Massachusetts is one of the states with the highest rates of health insurance coverage and most extensive health safety net for the poor. Evidence of this was clear in the decreased frequency and shorter duration of our Boston families' lapses in health care coverage. However, the more generous coverage did not entirely prevent periods with no insurance, nor did it address the lack of coverage for serious ongoing conditions. Our sampling design, including the selection of families with income at no more than 200 percent of the FPL, meant that in Boston we did not include families just over the threshold for some Medicaid coverage, those that would have been the most likely to experience periods with no medical coverage.

Prior to 1998, Illinois did not extend Medicaid eligibility beyond the federal requirement, covering children up to age six in families with incomes below 133 percent of the FPL and children up to age sixteen in families with incomes below the FPL. The state also covered teenagers in destitute households, which includes those with incomes below 50 percent of the FPL. Illinois' SCHIP program, KidCare, began in 1998 and expanded the number of eligible children in families with incomes below 133 percent of the FPL. At the time of the study, all children under nineteen years of age in these families were covered. Infants under one year old were covered in families with incomes up to 200 percent of the FPL. Illinois has a program for the medically needy to assist low- to moderate-income families that incur large medical expenses. As a consequence, families in Illinois experienced shorter lapses in coverage than families in Texas and were covered for more ongoing conditions.

TABLE 4.1. *Focal Child and Caregiver's Insurance Status, Wave 1 (Percentages)*

Caregiver's Insurance Status	Focal Child's Insurance Status				
	Employer or Union	Private/ Military/Other	No Insurance	Medicaid	Row%
Employer or Union	62%	2%	22%	14%	19%
Private/Military/ Other	5%	40%	4%	50%	6%
No Insurance	10%	1%	84%	5%	11%
Medicaid	1%	2%	0.2%	97%	64%
Column%	14%	4%	14%	68%	100%

The Extent of Health Insurance Coverage in the Three Cities

Our three states differ in potentially significant ways in eligibility criteria as well as other aspects of their Medicaid and SCHIP programs. Table 4.1 presents information from the Three City Study survey on the health insurance coverage for the caregiver and the focal child for whom we have extensive information from the first wave. The table compares different combinations of insurance coverage for the caregiver, who is in the vast majority of cases the focal child's mother, and the focal child. The table shows, for example, that among those caregivers who were covered by an employer-sponsored plan (19 percent of the sample), 62 percent of focal children were also covered by that plan. On the other hand, 22 percent of those children had no coverage of any sort and 14 percent are on Medicaid. When the mother had some other form of nongovernmental insurance, 40 percent of the children were covered by that plan and half were on Medicaid. Among those mothers with no insurance, the vast majority of their children also had no insurance. Given our selection criteria for the age of the focal child, 0–4 or 10–14, many of the mothers were still covered by Medicaid, which covers pregnant and nursing women, and in those cases so were nearly all of the focal children.

As in other studies, a large percentage of children in the Three City Study had no insurance. But the risk of lacking insurance differed significantly for different racial and ethnic groups. Figure 4.1 compares the percentages of children in our sample who have no health insurance of any sort for the different racial and ethnic groups in the study. The most striking finding, and one that is consistent with most previous

TABLE 4.2. *Percentage of Children Covered by Medicaid*

Family Income Relative to Federal Poverty Line	All 3 Cities	Boston	Chicago	San Antonio
<100%	77%	82%	82%	64%
100–124%	58%	86%	59%	30%
125–149%	53%	63%	61%	35%
150–199%	34%	64%	35%	5%

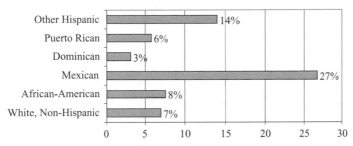

FIGURE 4.1. Percentage of children with no health insurance by race and Hispanic ethnicity

research, is the astonishingly high proportion of Mexican-origin children who have no coverage. Twenty-seven percent of the Mexican-origin children in our survey sample have no private or public coverage. For African Americans, this figure is 8 percent, and for non-Hispanic whites it is 7 percent. Clearly, this low rate of health insurance among Mexican-origin children represents a serious social problem. Even if these children receive charitable care or care from an emergency room, they do not have the one resource that might help assure continuity of care. These data make it clear that although in the United States we have a serious problem of lack of insurance among the poor, the problem is seriously confounded with aspects of race and Hispanic ethnicity.

In order to investigate the impact of state policy differences on Medicaid coverage, in Table 4.2 we present information on the proportion of children who were receiving Medicaid for different levels of family income expressed in terms of the ratio of family income to the federal poverty level (FPL). This table shows that while 77 percent of children in families with incomes below 100 percent of the FPL were covered in the sample as a whole, the proportion of children in these poorest families who were on Medicaid differed greatly among

TABLE 4.3. *Percentage of Focal Children and Caregivers Who Did Not Receive Needed Medical Care by City*

	City		
	Boston	Chicago	San Antonio
Focal Child	3%	5%	12%
Caregiver	7%	13%	18%

the three cities. Eighty-two percent of these children were covered in Boston and Chicago, but only 64 percent were covered in San Antonio. As family income increased, Medicaid coverage dropped in all three cities, but the drop was particularly pronounced in San Antonio. Among families with incomes between 150 percent and 200 percent of the FPL, only 5 percent of children were enrolled in San Antonio compared with 64 percent in Boston.

These city comparisons show how Medicaid coverage is related to state policy. At the time of the survey, Massachusetts had instituted the required and most of the optional coverage options provided by federal law. Texas, on the other hand, had not, resulting in the low coverage among families with incomes over 150 percent of the FPL, the income range in which states retained the greatest discretion as to whether to extend eligibility. These differences in coverage translated into differences in the use of health services. In the first wave of the survey, we asked respondents whether during the twelve months preceding the survey they had gone without health care they needed because they could not afford it. Table 4.3 shows that the percentage who reported going without needed care was higher for both the caregiver and the focal child in San Antonio than in Boston or Chicago. Boston's policy of maximizing coverage led to a lower proportion of caregivers who were forced to go without needed care in that city than in either of the two others.

State Medicaid Policies and Barriers to Health Care

Our study revealed three major barriers confronting low-income families in the struggle to get and keep health insurance in all three cities. The first barrier was the means-tested nature of public health insurance programs, for which one had to establish and reestablish eligibility.

Only families below certain income levels or those with slightly more income that include someone with a serious qualifying health problem could receive Medicaid. The second barrier arose from bureaucratic hurdles faced even by those families that were eligible for Medicaid. Families had to apply for each member of the household individually, recertify each one as required, and meet the constraints on "appropriate" use of medical services. In Chapter 3, for example, we introduced Darlence, who was threatened with reduced coverage if she continued to "overuse" her Medicaid by making the many appointments required by her complex medical conditions. The third barrier arose from difficulties families faced in locating a provider who would accept Medicaid even after they qualified, as well as securing transportation to that office or clinic. Given low Medicaid reimbursement rates and the bureaucratic effort required of providers, many physicians do not participate in the Medicaid program.

One might expect that as welfare policy, including that related to health care, has devolved to the states differences in how states choose to exercise their greater autonomy might mean that one's state of residence has a significant impact on the range and amount of health care a family receives. Although there have always been important elements of health care policy for the poor that have been determined at the state level, today states have even more control over the determination of eligibility, the nature and complexity of the application and recertification process, and the extent of services provided. Although states differ in their response to devolution, all state plans are still means-tested, bureaucratically complicated, and do not cover all conditions or all individuals and households in need.

In our study cities, as in cities across the nation, one's neighborhood, as well as the city and state, can affect the amount and type of health care available. A neighborhood with a free community health clinic or one with an emergency room that serves the neighborhood provides more opportunities for a poor family to get care than a neighborhood without such health care resources. In addition, transportation difficulties, especially in cities like San Antonio, which is widely spread out and has a poorly developed public transportation system, directly affect a family's access to health care, especially if they live far from available services. Helen, one of our San Antonio respondents, explained that her family owned a car even though they could hardly afford it. Car

ownership by families on welfare has been a long-standing criticism
of the system and often used in caricatures of welfare cheats, but in
cities that have been defined by the car and that have minimal public
transportation, the lack of an automobile can mean serious isolation.
Even though she owned a car, whenever possible Helen's family used
public transportation to get where they needed to go, including the doctor's office. There were times, however, such as when her daughter's
asthma became severe, that public transportation was just too slow and
inconvenient to be a viable option. For poor families that own a car,
social program asset tests can produce a veritable catch-22 because
ownership of a car worth over $2,000 can make a household ineligible
for some welfare programs. Ownership of a car often represents as
much of a burden as it does a useful asset. As our respondents pointed
out to us, cars that are worth less than $2,000 tend to be unreliable
and very expensive to operate.

Other geographic and neighborhood factors influence the availability of and access to health care as well. The size and layout of particular
neighborhoods can make a difference in and of itself. Western cities like
San Antonio are spread out over a large area. A block in San Antonio,
especially in residential areas, is usually much larger than a block in
Chicago or Boston. Neighborhoods and specific socioeconomic areas
within the city can be huge, as are the Mexican and African American
neighborhoods we studied. In San Antonio, distances from home to
work, to the supermarket, to school, to the day care center, to churches,
to the clinic, or to the welfare office can be great. The newer cities of
the West never developed subways or train systems, and their bus service to certain areas remains inadequate. In San Antonio, getting to
the welfare office, to work, or to the doctor on public transportation
often requires multiple bus transfers and several hours of travel time.
Many of our families in San Antonio, like Helen, used health care services that were on the other side of the city, and getting there and back
without a car could be an all-day ordeal. In Chicago and Boston, on
the other hand, neighborhoods are better-defined and less spread out.
Both cities have multiple forms of public transportation, and getting
around within the neighborhood and to other parts of the city is easier
than in San Antonio.

In all three cities, policy and ecology worked interactively and in conjunction with culture and economics defined the environment within

which families succeeded or failed in their attempts to obtain adequate health care. We must once again stress the point, however, that despite significant differences among the study cities, they all shared the characteristic that families faced difficulties in acquiring and maintaining health insurance for all household members. Differences in state policies and in access to health care were often overwhelmed by the basic welfare nature of Medicaid and other public programs. Means testing was universal, and applying for publicly funded health coverage always involved a bureaucratic process that was often poorly understood by those trying to use it.

In the End, the Similarities Outweigh the Differences

Very early in the study, it became obvious that the poor share certain similarities regardless of the state or city in which they live. In the survey component of the study, we found relatively few substantial city differences in the general socioeconomic profiles of families. In each city, residents of the poor neighborhoods that we studied had low levels of education, they were unemployed or worked at low-wage, unstable jobs, they frequently cycled on and off welfare, and they had irregular access to health care coverage, which they easily lost when they were able to obtain it. The caregivers in these families suffered from poor health, they had disrupted relationship and marital histories, and they experienced frequent and extended periods of unemployment. These patterns reflect a complex interaction of personal traits, specific racial and ethnic group histories of exclusion and discrimination, basic structural aspects of the U.S. economy and labor market, and the nature of our health care system. Of course, many of the similarities among our three samples arise from the fact that we intentionally selected them from poor neighborhoods defined in terms of high levels of disadvantage and need.

Despite what might seem like significant state-level differences in policy, all three cities share in the reality that the social welfare programs on which their inhabitants depend are based on the means-tested safety net approach characteristic of U.S. welfare policy in general. All state programs operate within federally mandated limits and can offer additional services only at their own expense. Most importantly, in all three cities, the reliance on public programs is stigmatizing. Rather than receiving health care as a citizenship right or as an employment benefit, those families that rely on Medicaid must reaffirm their pauper status on a regular basis in order to continue to receive services. As our interviews revealed, the recipients of publicly funded social services, including health services, live with the daily reality of sanctions, rejection, and humiliation. Although Massachusetts was more generous than Texas, Medicaid in Massachusetts, like food stamps or housing assistance, is a welfare program. In both states, it shares in the general problem of welfare for the poor, which is a fundamental problem for the nation at large.

In our opinion, there is no good welfare model for health care. Health care, like education, should be provided as a citizenship right because the collective welfare of the nation depends on the health of its people. If the United States had a universal and comprehensive health care financing system, states and localities would not differ based on state policy or on the basis of their population's ability to pay. Currently, states and localities do not differ greatly simply because all public health programs share the same characteristic of being programs for the poor, and all of them are increasingly responding to budgetary constraints and a growing public aversion to means-tested programs. For that reason, the situation in Texas shares with Massachusetts or Illinois more than might be readily apparent in terms of the problems that welfare recipients faced at the time of our research and are likely to face in the future. Again, we must reiterate that a focus on the experience of poor Texans at the welfare and Medicaid office tells us a story about national possibilities as all states deal with rising Medicaid budgets and serious budgetary shortfalls.

The Working Poor and the State Children's Health Insurance Program (SCHIP)

As Natalie's story illustrated, her application for Medicaid required multiple visits to the welfare office and considerable documentation for each individual for whom coverage was sought. During the period we worked in San Antonio, families were required to reestablish eligibility in person for each individual every six months, and they were often required to provide additional documentation at these times. For families with several children, families with children with serious health problems, or those in which parents had inflexible work schedules, the requirements for maintaining health insurance through Medicaid became serious obstacles both to continuous health coverage and employment. Legislative reforms have streamlined the application procedure to include mail-in applications and less frequent recertification requirements. During the time of the study, Texas, unlike the two other states, included assets in addition to income in the determination of Medicaid eligibility for children (Ross and Cox 2000).

All states currently operate an SCHIP program. Depending on each state's preference, its SCHIP program can consist of an extension of its Medicaid program, in which case it is required to offer the services offered under the Medicaid program, or it can consist of an entirely separate program that provides fewer services than Medicaid. During the time of our study, Texas' SCHIP plan had been approved but had just begun to enroll clients. In the two other states, the program was up and running. As with Medicaid, the eligibility criteria for SCHIP and the extent of the services covered differed among states. In Illinois, children in families with incomes at or below 185 percent of the FPL qualify for the program, whereas in Massachusetts and Texas the cutoff is 200 percent of the FPL. Although children in families with incomes up to 200 percent of the FPL qualify for SCHIP coverage in Texas, a large number of eligible children in that state are not enrolled, and in 2003 the state experienced a decline in enrollment so large that it resulted in an overall national decline even as thirty-seven other states had modest enrollment increases (Dunkelberg and O'Malley 2004; Smith, Rousseau, and O'Malley 2004).

Although states have the option of providing care to parents as part of their SCHIP program, as we shall see later, no public program covers the full range of health care needs of nondisabled working-age adults. In the United States, the primary route to health insurance is through employment, and as part of welfare reform and the new national mood, families are expected to leave welfare and become self-sufficient through work. Ideally, employment should provide health insurance coverage for the adult workers in the family as well as for the children. As we show in the next chapter, however, for workers at the bottom of the economic ladder, employment provides neither the wages that might make economic self-sufficiency possible nor the benefits that could replace the means-tested programs upon which poor families depend. As the cases we present in the next chapter show, because of the nature of the low-wage labor market and the highly restrictive participation criteria for many public programs, including those related to health, a family can find itself worse off once a parent goes to work than it was before.

5

Work and Health Insurance

A Tenuous Tie for the Working Poor

Despite the fact that most of the mothers on welfare we interviewed expressed a desire to work and to support themselves and their families, the reality of work in the low-wage service sector made self-sufficiency almost impossible. Many mothers in our study found that employment increased the difficulties they faced in maintaining a stable home life, and it frequently meant the loss of Medicaid. The objective of any rational welfare policy is to encourage work and to promote economic self-sufficiency and family stability. However, as we learned, in combination with the insecurities of low-wage work, the bureaucratic structures and rules that govern public support programs are often irrational and undermine the objectives they are intended to promote. In reality, few of our respondents were better off working than on welfare, yet most attempted to find employment whenever and wherever they could. Of course, as a result of welfare reform, they were required to do so, but most clearly would have preferred self-sufficiency over welfare dependency. The case of one young African American mother of four children illustrates many aspects of the work-related difficulties our respondents faced.

Sarah

Sarah, who we introduced in Chapter 2, had four children that ranged in age from three months to eight years. We conducted our initial interview in the family's small apartment, which was located in "The Courts," an old housing project close to downtown San Antonio.

During the interview, we were constantly interrupted by children shout-
ing and screaming, by incessant phone calls, by someone's changing of
television channels, and by the comings and goings of any number of
friends and relatives. Because of the heat, the windows had to remain
open, and construction work at the school across the street increased
the already high noise level that interfered with the flow of the conversation. All members of the family suffered from health problems, and
Sarah's unpredictable work schedule at a local social service agency
made it difficult to find time and energy to deal with them and the
many other problems that were a constant part of life at the edge. Like
so many other mothers in low-wage jobs, Sarah was required to work
a different number of hours from one week to the next and was never
quite sure what her schedule would be. Her job provided relatively
little income and no benefits.

The multiple demands of her life, in combination with the crowding
and noise at home, had clearly taken their toll on Sarah's emotional
health. When we first met her, she was tired and discouraged. Although
she was working and doing her best to become self-sufficient, she was
unable to establish the routines that might have introduced some predictability and stability into her family life. Because of her low income,
she was unable to move the family to better housing. According to
her, the family's apartment was in the worst section of the projects,
and she told us that "Most of the bad things in The Courts happen in
this area." In addition to her job and the demands of caring for her
children and maintaining the household, there were other demands on
Sarah's time and energy. Her mother, who was ill with diabetes, lived
about an hour and a half away by car. Although Sarah tried to offer
some assistance to the older woman, the distance and the fact that she
had no car made it difficult to visit or to provide the help her mother
needed. Periodically, she would take the bus to her mother's house, but
with four children the trip was expensive and tiring, and she often also
had to take time off work to make the trip.

At one point, Sarah's sister, who had three outstanding felony war-
rants and nowhere else to go, moved in with the family for a short
period. Just as she tried to help her mother, Sarah wanted to help her
sister, but in order to do so she ran the risk of being evicted if her sister's
presence was discovered. Her sister's presence not only added to the
practical burdens faced by the family but also increased the general

tension level of the household. The constant stress no doubt contributed to the family members' health problems, and these were a constant worry for Sarah. Three of the four children had asthma, and the fourth was born three months prematurely and suffered from other lingering respiratory problems that required ongoing medical attention. Sarah did her best to get the children the care they needed, but without health insurance from work she had to make difficult choices. When we met her, the children were being cared for by a pediatrician Sarah liked, but the doctor's office was on the other side of the city and it took an hour and a half to get there by bus. Conflicting work demands and the time it took to get to the doctor's office meant that Sarah avoided taking the children to the doctor unless it was absolutely necessary. As we mentioned in our introduction to Sarah, the children did not get routine care, nor was it clear that they were up on their inoculations. When the children developed serious symptoms, Sarah somehow managed to get them to the doctor.

The family's ability to get health care was made more difficult by Sarah's sense of pride and her determination not to use the emergency room or the public school system for health care. She insisted that the children get their shots at the doctor's office, where she had more control, instead of at school, where a local clinic occasionally made them available. One bright spot in Sarah's life resulted from the fact that her pediatrician went out of her way to help the family. At one point, when the family did not have Medicaid, the doctor worked with her on a payment schedule. Sarah was very appreciative and told us, "She's really good . . . like in one case, [she said] 'I'm sending somebody over there to come get you.' " The pediatrician sent someone to bring Sarah and the baby to the office because the doctor thought the child needed to be seen immediately.

Sarah herself had no health insurance throughout the entire study period. She had held six jobs in the three years preceding our interviews, but none provided health benefits. Although she told us that she enjoyed her current job at the social service agency, it clearly fell far short of providing for all of the family's needs. The fact that she liked the job and wanted to keep it placed her in a difficult situation. If she did not want to be fired, she could not take off from work for the appointments required to apply for, and then periodically reestablish, each child's eligibility for Medicaid. At one point, the family had been dropped from Medicaid completely because Sarah had missed too many appointments. Because she had no other choice, Sarah finally made the work and income sacrifice required to apply for Medicaid, but the effort was not successful. Even though she kept her appointment, her application was denied because she failed to bring some supporting documentation. In order to avoid skipping work to bring the additional documentation to the Medicaid office, Sarah faxed the documentation from her job, but the fax was not accepted and her application was again denied.

At one point, when times got really hard, Sarah applied for emergency assistance, which, as she understood it, provided short-term support to those not on TANF. This program provided assistance with rent and with transportation expenses, but it did not address the family's health care coverage problems because it did not include eligibility for Medicaid. For Sarah, the need to seek such aid was humiliating; she felt that the caseworker did not believe her and even implied that she was not a good mother. She told us that the caseworker asked "Well how did you go four months without food stamps, Medicaid, or a job? How do you pay your bills?" Lacking any power or influence when confronting the bureaucracy, Sarah had no choice but to endure whatever the process meted out. As she said, "Every time you go in there it's a different change they've made. You spend a whole day down there. They want to know how many men, especially when you're doing the child support papers, man, how many times [you've had sex]! I mean it's so personal."

The confusion and difficulty that were part of applying for welfare and health insurance mirrored themselves in many other areas of the family's life. Work, rather than providing solutions to the family's problems, only complicated them. Sarah lived in a world of bureaucratic rules and regulations in which she was not an influential client to be courted and shown respect but rather a powerless pauper who had to beg for information and help from an intractable and unsympathetic system. Her job gave her no power or social standing. Her attempts to find better housing were a constant struggle and another example of the complexities of the bureaucratic system that she had to negotiate. The family had been on the waiting list for "Section 8" housing, the major housing subsidy program for the poor, for nine years. However, Sarah did not actually understand how the waiting list worked or that she had to reconfirm her interest on a regular basis. When she failed to do so, she was dropped from the list, and when she finally called the Housing Authority to inquire about her position in the queue, she learned that she was no longer on the list at all.

Like all low-wage parents, Sarah had few resources, whether in terms of time, energy, or money, with which to deal with the demands of work and the requirements of the Medicaid bureaucracy or other parts of the welfare system. The demands that the combination of work and family life placed on her were often overwhelming and always demoralizing. During the last few months that we were in contact with the family, neither Sarah nor her children had health insurance. Her attempts to obtain coverage remained an ongoing struggle. For families like Sarah's, a successful application for Medicaid for one child can represent only a temporary victory. The coverage is by no means permanent, and because Medicaid does not offer full family coverage, each child must be qualified separately. Sarah's job could not provide her with the benefits or wages she needed. It was clear that she paid a penalty for her efforts to comply with her own and society's expectation that she work and attempt to support herself and her family. The problem, as our data reveal, lies in the structure of the low-wage employment market, which makes escape from poverty difficult and potentially undermines the health of children and adults. We will revisit Sarah later in this chapter.

Work Is Not Enough Even When You Can Get It

The families in our study provided many insights into just how weak the tie between work and health care coverage is for so many adults and children in the United States. Although most middle-class Americans have employer-based health insurance that covers all members of the family, those at the bottom of the income and occupational hierarchies, a population that like our sample is disproportionately African American and Hispanic, find themselves at best with episodic coverage or coverage for only some members of the family and at worst without any coverage at all. The families in our study were rarely offered employer-based insurance, a fact that was of little real consequence because few could have afforded the required employee contribution out of their low wages. Yet when they found work they faced a serious

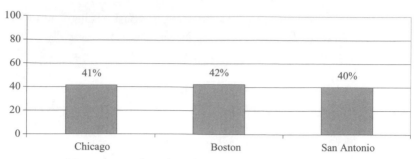

FIGURE 5.1. Percentage of employed primary caregivers by city

dilemma. Even relatively low wages could place at least some members of the family above the eligibility threshold for Medicaid. Two-parent families in which both parents work were at particularly high risk of losing eligibility.

The new State Children's Health Insurance Program (SCHIP) clearly addresses part of the problem but does not solve it. As we documented in Chapter 4, many eligible children remain uncovered, and the SCHIP program does not generally cover adults. Individuals without health insurance do not, of course, go without health care altogether because many federal and state programs and some local programs provide care to individuals without private coverage (Bauman and Herrick 2000). These programs, however, are still charity, and they often have restrictive eligibility requirements. They rarely provide all of the care individuals or families need, especially for chronic care or mental illness, nor do charitable sources provide the continuous and seamless care that the middle class enjoys and expects.

As our ethnographic interviews revealed, tenuous and weak ties to the labor force, episodic and discontinuous employment, and jobs in the service sector placed employment-based coverage out of the reach of all but a small fraction of our study families. Only a very small fraction of our respondents worked full-time. Figure 5.1 shows that in fact only about 40 percent of the respondents in the survey reported that they had worked at all for pay during the past week in any of the three cities. The ethnography made it clear that these survey-based figures included individuals who were working part-time as well as those who were only temporarily employed and who would lose their jobs the following week. Some of those who reported not working last week would find work the next week. In light of the volatility in the

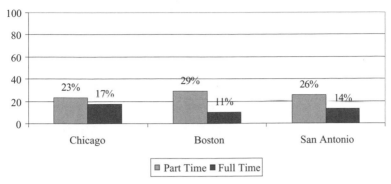

FIGURE 5.2. Type of employment for primary caregivers by city

employment status of this population, it is clear that snapshots of the sort we get from surveys tell an incomplete story and that the distinction between employed and unemployed is imprecise for the working poor. Many of the working poor have low incomes because they work only part-time, either voluntarily or because they do not have the option of working more hours. Among our respondents, part-time work was the only employment that most could find. Figure 5.2 presents information on the number of hours the respondent usually worked each week. Most respondents did not work at all, and in Figure 5.2 we differentiate between those who reported that they usually worked between one and thirty-nine hours per week and those who reported that they usually worked forty hours or more. It was up to the respondent, of course, to interpret what the term "usual" meant. The question did not refer to last week and could have been interpreted as how much one works in one's current job, one's last job, or even how much one would like to work.

However the respondents interpreted the question, the figure shows that the employment experiences of parents in the three cities were fairly similar. Less than 30 percent of the three samples reported that they usually worked between one and thirty-nine hours. An even lower proportion reported working full-time or more. Between approximately 10 percent and 17 percent of respondents reported that they worked forty or more hours. The fact that respondents reported slightly more part-time work and slightly less full-time work in Boston than in the two other cities may again reflect Massachusetts's more liberal welfare policies. Regardless of city, however, it is clear that regular

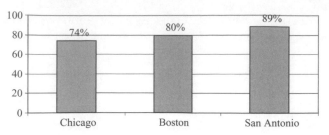

FIGURE 5.3. Percentage of primary caregivers employed in the services sector by city

employment was not the norm among the respondents in the survey. These statistics reveal low rates of employment but do not tell the whole story, which was one characterized by much instability and churning in and out of the labor force and between jobs. These statistics, in fact, probably overstate the real employment status of our respondents.

As these data illustrate, one of the core problems with employment-based health coverage for the working poor results from the fact that employers in the low-wage service sector frequently offer an employee only part-time work with variable hours and rarely offer health insurance. Given their low profit margins, employers in the service sector often cannot afford to offer coverage to their employees. Even outside the service sector, low-wage workers are far less likely than better-paid workers to have health insurance (Claxton et al. 2004; Collins et al. 2003).

Figure 5.3 shows that the vast majority of those respondents in the survey who worked did so in the service sector, which includes jobs in areas such as fast food, retail, general health, and maintenance. Some workers in this sector worked informally as housekeepers, child care workers, babysitters, volunteers, and community workers. Again, some city differences emerge from the survey. A larger percentage of workers in San Antonio, for example, were employed in services than in either Chicago or Boston. For the most part, however, the jobs our respondents held in each city were not very different. Data from the ethnography also revealed that the jobs that parents held were similar in all three cities and included domestic work, clerical work, child care, fast food and cafeteria work, and work in other service occupations and for temporary agencies. In each city, a handful of women found more stable employment, but they were the exception. One

San Antonio mother was a bank clerk and one Chicago mother worked for a management company. A few others held such jobs, but most did not.

Boston presents an interesting picture. As in Chicago and San Antonio, a substantial fraction of parents in Boston had been unemployed for a long period, if they had in fact ever worked. Most of the jobs our respondents in Boston held were similar to those held by our Chicago and San Antonio respondents. However, seven of the mothers in the Boston ethnographic sample reported jobs that seemed from their descriptions to promise real employment stability and security. However, upon closer examination of the circumstances of each of these cases, it was clear that the stability was only apparent and these cases illustrate why this slightly elevated tier of jobs did not offer any real long-term security. One mother had acquired the skills and contacts to obtain a full-time job as a receptionist at the time we first met her. However, we found out that she had worked at four different jobs in the preceding two years. Each job had been interrupted by a combination of family illness and child care problems that made it necessary for her to quit working. Like the mothers in clearly inferior jobs, she had no backup or reserve with which to weather the crises even once she had found a better job.

Another Boston mother worked between thirty and forty hours per week as a cell phone technician. However, her job provided no benefits, and she was vulnerable to the problems that any illness that she or her children might experience could cause. A third mother held a full-time job in a medical records office, but after a year and a half she still had no benefits and was also vulnerable to health crises. A fourth mother worked in a hospital kitchen. She had some health benefits, but her salary remained so low that she was dependent on both subsidized housing and food stamps.

Three other Boston mothers seemed to enjoy real job stability. One worked as a medical assistant at a job that provided family health benefits. The two others worked as a bank teller and for a major hotel chain. Two of these women had some college education, but what really seemed to make a difference was the fact that they shared housing with another person who provided full-time child care. Even for these women, however, employment stability could not be taken for granted. The hotel chain worker had begun working when her youngest child entered elementary school. The school offered an extended day care program that made it possible for her to work, and she had been working for a fairly long period. Unfortunately, when tourism in Boston took a downturn, she was laid off. When we were last in contact with her, she was living on unemployment insurance that would soon end, and her health insurance had been terminated.

The medical assistant was taking classes at a local community college and hoped to become a licensed registered nurse in a year or two. Her dream was to move to Florida, where, as she said, "there's a good community for the kids, where the rent is good, and where the pay is good, where they have lots of hospitals and they'll have opportunities for me." Completing her education and qualifying as a professional was clearly her route to self-sufficiency, but it was a route few mothers could make work. The bank teller, who was Latina and had an excellent command of both English and Spanish, received a promotion to customer service representative and was transferred to a new suburban branch. There, however, she was the only Hispanic and had serious difficulties with her supervisor, who criticized her language skills and even made reference to her ethnicity. The situation was clearly strained, and she received an unsatisfactory performance evaluation, which she refused to sign. As we shall see in the next chapter, for minority Americans the fact of race and ethnicity often affects their employment opportunities and experiences. After speaking to the personnel manager and a vice president at the bank, she was able to move back to her original branch, although she was afraid that even though her recent performance evaluations had been good, the bad performance evaluation she had received from the previous supervisor would hurt her chances for further promotions.

These women, even with their employment insecurities, were clearly the exception. We fairly quickly came to realize that even among those who claimed to be employed, many worked at jobs that were in reality informal and unstable. Many in fact really stretched the meaning of the term "job." The work they took provided low and unpredictable wages and no benefits. Many middle-class families routinely employ cleaning ladies and gardeners and pay them in cash. Neither the employer nor the employee pays Social Security or other taxes. Such jobs are quite common in our economy and were common among our ethnographic respondents. The fact that our respondents were so often unclear about

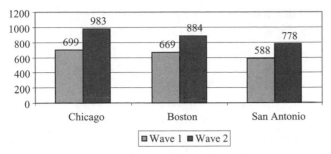

FIGURE 5.4. Average monthly income for working primary caregiver by city

their employment and insurance situations leads us to suspect that survey reports of employment and amount of work performed by those at the economic margin contain substantial misinformation. Such error again reflects the ambiguity and instability in the work lives of the working poor.

States, of course, differ in their labor market compositions, their wage rates, and other aspects of employment, and we wondered whether these differences might have an impact on the earnings of our study families. Figure 5.4 shows that in both waves of the survey total household earnings were higher in Chicago than in Boston and lowest in San Antonio. By the second wave of the survey, after welfare reform had forced some individuals to find jobs, average monthly earnings in San Antonio were less than $800 a month. An income of $800 a month translates into annual earnings of $9,600. In Chicago, where earnings were nearly $1,000 a month, average annual earnings still totaled only $12,000. In 2001, the federal poverty level for a single mother with two children was $14,269. Clearly, earnings at this level are too low to allow a family to become self-sufficient, and even slightly increased earnings place a working poor family at risk of losing the means-tested benefits that its members so desperately need.

These data then clearly illustrate the dilemma that low-wage families face. The earnings they receive from the jobs they can find leave them with no discretionary income with which to purchase expensive private health care coverage. Yet their desire to work and the requirements of welfare reform force them into jobs that may jeopardize their family's health care coverage. As we have noted, the national statistics on the number of Americans without health insurance are disturbing in and of themselves, but they cannot convey the complexity and urgency of the real-life situations that poor and working-class families face as a result of the instability of their medical care coverage and the resulting variability in their access to health care. A large body of research clearly documents the fact that the lack of health insurance reduces health care use by individuals and results in poorer health (Institute of Medicine 2002a). Poor health reduces one's productivity and long-term career opportunities. The lack of health insurance therefore has major long-term individual and social implications. Our interviews revealed that the instability in health coverage is both the result of instability in work and also one aspect of the work lives of working poor families that creates and perpetuates family instability. The stories we recount in this chapter reveal how elusive middle-class stability is for the poor, especially in terms of health care coverage.

Marginal workers, including many employed single mothers, have never enjoyed health care security for themselves or their children. Medicaid and SCHIP represent clear improvements that, at least in theory, address many of the health care financing problems of the working poor, at least for their children. However, the mothers in our study experienced the impact of several trends that during the last decade have changed the nature of the jobs available to them and have made employment even less stable. These trends have often left employed mothers with less access to health insurance coverage for themselves, and to some extent their children, than unemployed mothers. Single mothers, especially those with low levels of education, have historically had considerable difficulty in finding and keeping well-paid full-time employment. The demands of child care and employment often conflict, and much of the work available to young women is seasonal or unpredictable because of the volatility of the markets within which many service-sector employers operate.

Only a small proportion of the mothers in our ethnography remained employed for long periods in jobs with regular hours. For the most part, when mothers were employed, they held jobs that did not include even a rudimentary benefit package. Women and their children were not only ineligible for employer-assisted health insurance but also rarely entitled to the sick days or personal days that would allow them to retain their jobs when the mother or child became seriously ill. Finally, even when mothers found full-time employment in jobs that offered health coverage, they could rarely afford either the employee contribution required or the co-payments that were required for office visits and prescriptions. Their access to dental care and eye care was often determined by their very limited access to some form of charitable or discounted service.

In exploring the work–health insurance nexus, or rather the lack of it, for our ethnographic families more closely, we begin with an analysis of their basic employment patterns and difficulties and illustrate the extent to which their experience is dominated by episodic and marginal jobs. We also examine the extent and nature of employer-provided benefit packages to which a service-sector worker might have access and illustrate the numerous reasons that they do not take advantage of such coverage even when it is offered. Finally, we explore the alternatives that low-income mothers often turn to when they or their children need medical care.

Employed or Not

An initial review of the most recent jobs held by the mothers in the ethnography provides insights into the survey findings of very low employment rates and reveals the difficulties that marginal workers face in finding and holding jobs. Our initial coding of the 155 ethnographic families (from all three cities) for which we had the most complete job information revealed that approximately one-third (56) were unemployed for a period of at least several months prior to our interviews (Lein et al. 2005). Of the remaining two-thirds, only about one-third (33 of 99) held a single, nearly full-time job. These jobs were predominantly in the service sector and included work in health services, food preparation and serving, domestic work, and sales. Even those mothers who worked close to full-time experienced some shift in hours worked, and few had access to affordable benefits. The handful of mothers with full-time employment and benefits that included at least some health care coverage held manufacturing jobs or jobs in public service. Only one mother in our San Antonio ethnographic sample received health care benefits that covered the entire family through work. Through diligence and hard work, this mother had advanced in the organization for which she worked and had finally arrived at her current position, but she continued to worry about what would happen to her family should her employer go out of business or were she to lose her job.

The rest of the women in our sample pieced together multiple jobs, were often underemployed and worked only part-time involuntarily, and experienced frequent spells of unemployment. This work instability and unpredictability undermined any attempt they made to develop routines and to organize their daily lives, let alone gain skills and experience that would allow them to seek different kinds of work. Some of our mothers worked continuously but were constantly underemployed, and we came to realize that given the nature of marginal work, underemployment is in many ways far worse than unemployment, especially as it often affects eligibility for public programs. These underemployed women earned poverty-level wages but they were, particularly in Texas, ineligible for welfare assistance or public health insurance.

The work lives of the families we interviewed were unstable in all three cities, and a parent's employment affected Medicaid eligibility in each. The higher eligibility ceiling for Medicaid in Illinois and Massachusetts compared with Texas meant that more mothers and children remained eligible while mothers were employed in those two cities. In all three cities, however, mothers still lost their eligibility before their children did, and in all three cities jobs and medical insurance were jeopardized by the demands of the Medicaid application and recertification process. Sarah, the young African American mother with whose story we began the chapter, had to struggle constantly with the unpredictability that work imposed on her life and on her access to health care.

More of Our Interactions with Sarah

Sarah's situation was typical of that of the other families in our study and illustrates the extent of discontinuity in her employment and her family's health care coverage. As in the majority of the other cases, the combination of the unpredictability of her employment and difficulties with the recertification process resulted in interruptions in coverage. Sarah's case, however, introduced a new complication that made her situation even more difficult. Sarah was involved in an abusive relationship that finally made it necessary for her to move in order to escape her abusive partner. As a result of the move, both her work and the family's Medicaid coverage were again interrupted.

When Sarah's three older children were infants, the family was on TANF and Medicaid, although her coverage was not continuous.

TABLE 5.1. *Time Line of Sarah's Employment and Health History in 2000*

The Year 2000	1st Quarter	2nd Quarter	3rd Quarter	4th Quarter
Job	Working at day care center	Meat-packing job	Clerical work	Clerical work at child care facility
Health Insurance – Self	Medicaid	None	None	None
Health Insurance – Children	Medicaid	None	None	Medicaid
Health Problems	Child with respiratory ailment	Child with respiratory ailment	Child with respiratory ailment; daughter has burn	Child with respiratory ailment; son develops small tumor

Sarah remained with her children's father through this period, and the fact that he was in the household and had earnings affected the family's eligibility because the family income criteria are less generous for older children and the spouse's income, even if low, adds to the household total. Just before Thanksgiving in 1999, the relationship deteriorated and she called the police after a fight that was provoked by his treatment of her children. The initial argument escalated into a serious fight and he beat her. When the police arrived, they arrested him and he was jailed, after which he was placed on parole. Around Christmas, he called her, but when she hung up on him he came to the house in a rage and beat her again. As a result, his probation was revoked and he went back to jail.

The first jail sentence and period of parole sent the family into a very chaotic year. In order to attempt to make sense of the very complex narrative of the events of that year, we present it in Table 5.1 as a time line that summarizes Sarah's employment status, her health insurance status, the health insurance coverage of her children, and their health problems, as she related them. While working in turn at the day care center and the clerical jobs, Sarah was able to negotiate for the time she needed to recertify her children for Medicaid. She herself was not eligible for Medicaid while she was working, but none of the jobs she held offered health insurance so she went without any coverage. During her time at the meat-packing plant, however, the entire family was dropped from Medicaid because Sarah missed appointments for recertification. She could not take time off work because of the loss of pay and the risk that she would be fired for excessive absences. As the direct consequence of policies that are designed to encourage mothers toward employment, the mothers themselves often face trade-offs between employment and health insurance.

The narratives provided by our respondents were complicated and, as in Sarah's case, they did not always make sense and did not always offer clear sequences of events or plausible justifications or explanations for what happened. The reasons for the frequent job transitions, for example, were not always obvious, nor might they have been entirely clear to the respondents themselves. Sarah told us, for example, that she left the job in the day care center for the better pay and more regular hours at the meat-packing plant. However, she then left that job for the clerical job because she needed more flexibility in order to meet the demands of the welfare system and have the greater freedom to apply for health insurance and child care benefits for her children. Without a child care subsidy, and with her aunt unable to care for her children full-time, Sarah changed jobs yet again to work at a day care center where her children could accompany her. She was able to negotiate enough flexibility in that job to allow her to make the necessary appointments to regain Medicaid for her children.

During the following year, her children's father, in jail for attacking her, threatened to find her and hurt her when he was released. To escape from him, in 2001, just as we ended our data collection, she moved to a different city and started her life over, including new attempts to find employment and obtain health insurance. Sarah spent a great deal of time and effort to obtain and maintain Medicaid eligibility for her children, and these struggles interacted with the difficulties of finding and keeping a job as well as supervision and care of her children. Her case also illustrates how few options adults have for health care insurance for themselves. Both the ethnographic data and the survey data show that a much higher proportion of children than parents have health insurance. Gloria, whose story follows, illustrates the difficulties faced by caregivers who cannot find health coverage for themselves, even when they can keep their children insured.

TABLE 5.2. *Time Line of Gloria's Employment and Health History,*
1999–2001

	1999	2000	2001
Jobs	Works at hamburger restaurant; cleans motel rooms; works at family restaurant	Works at hamburger restaurant	Works at family restaurant
Health Problems	Falls at work/breaks arms; children face series of illnesses; takes children out of day care	Loses child care subsidy	Shares child care with her partner

Gloria

The situation of another young non-Hispanic white mother further illustrates the complex tie between unstable work, an unstable family life, and unstable health care coverage even for nonminority families. It also illustrates the hopelessness of Gloria's attempt to obtain health care for herself. While Gloria was trying hard to make sure her children had health insurance, she simply did without it herself. As a result, she was forced to manage her own health care differently from that of her children. Gloria was twenty-two years old when we met her. She had a three-year-old girl and two-year-old twin boys. The girl and the twins had different fathers. The father of the twins was in another relationship and had not visited his children in over a year. The older child's father, however, was still involved and visited the little girl and made occasional financial contributions to the family. All three children had been diagnosed with asthma, and one of the twins was developmentally delayed. Because they were so young, the children had been covered by Medicaid almost continuously since their births, except for a few lapses when the recredentialing process did not go smoothly. Gloria never had health insurance. As a result, and as we will explain in greater detail, when she suffered a work-related accident that required medical care, she had to go to court to try to get payment from her employer in order to cover the costs of her treatment.

As in Sarah's case, Gloria's life is complicated and her account sometimes rambling, so we summarize the highlights in the three-year time line in Table 5.2. Gloria left high school after the tenth grade. She worked in fast food restaurants for several years and was in one of those jobs when her first child was born. However, because of a combination of health problems and child care problems, she was unable to hold on to any one job for long and moved from one service-sector job to another, experiencing ongoing intermittent unemployment.

Each work transition was marked by some problem related, at least in part, to difficulties in obtaining health care or arranging for child care. In 1999, Gloria, as usual, had no health insurance and suffered the job-related injury we mentioned earlier. She was then unable to continue at the job on which she was injured and searched for a new job at the same time she was involved in legal action that she hoped would result in a court judgment forcing her employer to pay for her work-related medical expenses. Before she was fully recovered, she took a job cleaning motel rooms. She was able to accept the job offer because at that time she qualified for and was able to find subsidized child care. Her employment problems and the family's health problems continued, however. All three children suffered a series of infections, and Gloria lost the cleaning job because of her absences from work that resulted from the children's health problems. She then spent a few months unemployed.

Determined to work, Gloria found another fast food job and worked there until she felt that the subsidized day care program that she had been using was not taking adequate care of her children, particularly when they were ill. Perhaps because they were not getting adequate care, or because of the other stresses in their lives, the children's health was deteriorating, and when their chronic health problems became serious, Gloria was unable to send them to regular child care. As a result, Gloria lost her child care subsidy. Because finding and paying for child care for three children herself was impossible, Gloria was forced to reconsider her strategies. In her next job, the fast food job she had when we last interviewed her, she worked a late shift so that she could care for the children during the day. While she worked, her new partner stayed home with the children.

In spite of all her difficulties finding and keeping a job, Gloria believed that work was important and that it was much better for her children for her to work than for the family to be on welfare. Throughout the period during which we were in contact with her, she remained diligent in her attempts to stay employed. Despite her determination, however, health and other family problems overcame her best efforts, and even though she intensely disliked being on welfare, occasionally it could not be avoided. Even the need to apply for Medicaid was demeaning to her. "It [dealing with Medicaid] is difficult because they never trust you and every time you go you have to prove you don't have a car, what your income is, and that you don't have any other bank accounts." Gloria was typical of mothers who found themselves facing a number of bureaucratic obstacles in their search for health care even though it was self-evident that publicly supported health insurance was their only possible recourse.

Gloria's access to health care was reduced because she worked. She was ineligible for Medicaid, but her job offered no health benefits. Her children were eligible for Medicaid, but the work required to keep them continuously covered put her jobs at risk. Furthermore, as her children get older, their eligibility for Medicaid will decline, again especially if Gloria continues to work. Indeed, if Gloria, or any of the other women in our study, were to actually succeed in increasing their incomes, they would probably end up worse off from a health insurance standpoint because of the loss of Medicaid or SCHIP. During one interview, Gloria told us that she intended to apply for the low-payment reduced cost and debt management program we mentioned earlier that is intended for people who are not eligible for Medicaid. Gloria realized that, working or not, she had to accept some help; however, the reduced payment program is not an entitlement program. Its ability to help is limited by its funds, and it was unclear whether Gloria succeeded in receiving that service. With three children who are chronically ill, she continued to combine work with ongoing recertification for Medicaid for her children. Gloria's own income kept her above any eligibility for Medicaid for herself, and her other options were limited.

Gloria's determination to be a responsible parent and her concern with health care, with work, and with child care were motivated by her desire to be a better parent than her own mother. Like almost all of the other women we talked with in the course of our study, Gloria's core identity was that of mother, and all of her other roles and activities were defined by and supported that core identity. Gloria was one of thirteen children and as she explained, "There were just too many of us. . . . I want to spend more quality time with them [her own children]. . . . I want to let them know that they can talk to me instead of learning everything on the street like I did." On top of her struggles to earn a living, to maintain health coverage at least for her children, and to locate responsible child care, Gloria also worried that she could not spend the time necessary with her children to do a good job raising them. Like many of the struggling mothers we interviewed, Gloria's parental role was undermined by the characteristics of the service-sector jobs she held.

The Service-Sector Trap

The problems that our ethnographic families experienced are becoming more common in general because as in our study cities manufacturing jobs are being displaced by low-wage service-sector jobs in the nation as a whole (Bivens, Scott, and Weller 2003; Bluestone and Harrison 1988; Bureau of Labor Statistics 2004a; Bureau of Labor Statistics 2004b; Congressional Budget Office 2004; Didrickson 1997; Thompson 1999). Workers with low levels of education and experience, and the women we interviewed in particular, are very unlikely to find unionized manufacturing jobs that include guarantees of hours, wages, and benefits. Like Gloria, they are more likely to find work in food services, health care, and retail sales in which union organization, especially in right-to-work states such as Texas, has been unsuccessful.

Except for young workers who hold service jobs while they finish their education or for temporary purposes, few service-sector jobs are part of a career ladder. The work histories of the older mothers in our sample illustrate how one service job follows another, each with similarly low wages and no access to health insurance. Thus, although the relatively short-term "transition" benefits are often available to families as they depart welfare, they only delay the almost inevitable arrival of a time when at least some members of the household will lose health insurance coverage when a parent becomes a wage earner. One of the older mothers in the ethnographic study, Dora, had been in and out of the labor force since 1989, when she began her work life in a jewelry store after high school. Dora stopped working shortly after her second child was born, so that she could stay home to care for her two children. At the time, she was still married, but when she separated from her husband in 1994, she was forced to take a job at a fast food restaurant that she found through a referral from friends. She worked at that job for three months and then switched to a job at a buffet restaurant, where she worked for another nine months. Neither job offered benefits, and both had rotating shifts.

Dora received TANF for several years after the birth of her second child until she resumed restaurant work as a waitress for a year. In a rather short period, she moved from the waitress job to a bookstore job and then to a job at a grocery store. None of these job transitions resulted in a substantial improvement in Dora's situation. In none of her jobs was she employed full-time or offered benefits. When the study ended, Dora had left the grocery store job because her child care arrangements, which were always a bit irregular, fell through. When we were last in contact with her, she was in the process of rearranging child care and trying to get back into the labor market. Like so many of our mothers who had only a high school education and few job skills, the low-wage service sector provided no access to improved wages, stability, or skills. At various points, her children's medical coverage lapsed, and Dora herself was usually without health insurance. Workers in this sector have very little hope of ever obtaining health care coverage for themselves or their children through work.

Unpredictable Schedules

These cases illustrate the extent of instability in our respondents' job histories. Jobs in the low-wage service sector require few skills and are easy to get and easy to lose. Most of our respondents had held many such jobs, and their narratives made it clear that one of the characteristics of such jobs that undermines stability is the worker's lack of control over his or her work schedule. Our respondents had little control over their schedules, the number of hours they worked, their earnings, or any other aspects of their jobs. Our interviews revealed just how unpredictable the daily schedules of low-wage workers can be and how that unpredictability undermines their attempts to get ahead. This instability of work itself is a very poorly understood aspect of low-wage employment that results in what might be seen as irresponsible behavior or a lack of initiative on the part of workers themselves.

Work schedules that change from week to week make it almost impossible to enroll in training programs or to piece together additional jobs that might allow a poorly educated, low-income parent to develop work-related skills or to increase his or her earnings. Even if a mother has free hours one week, she may have to work during those times the next week. That lack of predictability affects the whole family and interacts with problems maintaining health care coverage. A less than full-time job that offers no benefits, sick leave, or vacation days can become full-time in its effects. The result is a catch-22 in which low-wage work provides no valuable job skills and keeps a worker from increasing his or her human capital through education or from earning extra income through additional work. These families find that their health care benefits are often as unstable as their jobs. Although children may regain access to Medicaid during periods of parental unemployment, such coverage requires considerable time and energy to maintain and rarely extends to the unemployed adults in the family.

Work by a team of researchers in Chicago documents the ways in which the growing number of service-sector jobs in which our mothers are likely to work are structured to prevent those who work in them from gaining the status of full-time employees or becoming self-sufficient (Lambert, Waxman, and Haley-Lock 2002). Like our ethnographic data, this research shows that although such jobs may have set hourly wage rates, the number and scheduling of hours worked vary from week to week and are not under the control of the employee. As a consequence, one's income varies, sometimes dramatically, and scheduling, budgeting, and saving are difficult. One spends virtually all of what one earns for daily needs, and any meager savings one manages to put away can be easily wiped out by an emergency or during a period of underemployment or unemployment.

Jobs in health services, fast food, and retail often schedule their employees for one week at a time. Although individuals who hold these jobs may be classified as full-time workers, they seldom work a full thirty-five to forty hours a week and do not receive the predictable income of true full-time workers. Unpredictable schedules make it almost impossible to enroll in training programs or to piece together additional jobs. The result is a situation in which low-wage work provides little stability, few valuable job skills, and keeps a woman from acquiring additional human capital through education or additional income through additional work.

No Job Security

Many of the jobs the mothers in our ethnographic sample worked were short-term. In many cases, the work was seasonal or the jobs were dependent on the high end of a business cycle. Often the work was sufficiently physically demanding that most workers could only tolerate the job for a limited amount of time. Again, however, the common denominator was that workers in these jobs had little security and were unable to negotiate wage levels or the hours they worked. In these environments, negotiating for benefits was hardly an option. Much of this powerlessness came from the nature of the jobs and the fact that they were relatively easy to get and easy to lose. Jobs in agriculture, the tourist industry, public schools, and other work domains are often seasonal, and low-wage workers are often laid off or offered only short-term contracts. The mothers in our sample were clearly part of the growing sector of contingent employees who are hired when extra help is needed and let go when that need ends.

The instability at work and low wages, along with the lack of benefits, result in and interact with other uncertainties in families' lives in ways that make it even more difficult for a parent to keep a job. A parent's own illness or injury, a child's sickness or disability, the requirements of the welfare system for frequent recertification, and a host of other problems interfered with many mothers' ability to remain employed. Most of the marginal jobs in which our mothers worked did not provide sick days or personal days, and very frequently a short absence because of illness or some other family emergency meant termination.

A Last Visit with Sarah

Sarah, who held the twenty-hour "full-time" job described earlier, was ineligible for benefits on that job because of its hourly nature. In order to make ends meet, she also took care of her friend's child for thirteen hours a week. Because she had no alternative, she turned to the public health care system for her children but remained uninsured herself. Her wages placed her well above the extremely low income

threshold for adult women. Because one of her children had respiratory problems, Sarah had applied for SSI for the child, but that application was denied. Meanwhile, she had no insurance for herself, and
her struggles to maintain it for her children continued.

Sarah's case illustrates many of the health insurance problems that
our mothers faced once they entered the labor force. In general, the
jobs they were able to find did not offer health insurance. As we noted
in Chapter 1, employment-based health insurance coverage expanded
rapidly after the Second World War but seems to have reached a satu-
ration point. Even jobs that pay far more than those our respondents
qualified for no longer offer the low-cost health insurance they once
provided employees (Claxton et al. 2004; Collins et al. 2003). The costs
of health care and health care coverage have skyrocketed. Employers
have no choice but to pass a larger fraction of the cost on to their
employees or to drop health insurance altogether. There is little reason
to believe that the situation will become anything but worse for low-
wage workers as employers continue to limit coverage or pass more of
the cost on to employees and as the federal and state budgets for health
care are curtailed by austerity measures.

Conclusion: Work Is Not Enough

One aspect of the lives of the poor that became obvious to us during
our study and that we will explore in greater depth in the next
chapter was the extent to which the hopelessness of the reality of
their situations came to define their expectations. Few mothers had
adequate incomes or any real chance of ever becoming self-sufficient,
and almost none had continuous health insurance. Self-sufficiency
and continuous household health care coverage were simply outside
of the realities of their lives. Although these women wished to work
and to be as responsible as they could in their roles as parents, they
held few expectations that work would greatly improve their lot.
In fact, the possibility of health insurance through employment was
so irrelevant to our respondents that they rarely mentioned it as a
factor in deciding which jobs they would take. Their decisions about
which job to accept or whether to work at all were based on more
rudimentary considerations such as which job was least onerous in
terms of hours, child care requirements, and location. Women in this
situation quickly become realists, and, as one mother candidly told us,

it is the nature of the work available to women like her that explains why so many mothers cycle off and on welfare.

Because when they get off welfare, they get a job at McDonald's because they have no education. As soon as they get a job, they lose their food stamps, they lose their Medicaid, and they have to start paying rent, insurance. They can't afford that. So they work for two months, then get off and go back on welfare. You have a year. Then you work a month or two, then get off and go back on welfare. You have another year. So it's almost the way they've learned to beat the system. Even now, at the program, you're supposed to work.

In the few cases where employer-sponsored health insurance was an option, mothers still had problems taking advantage of it. In a few cases, mothers were offered health insurance but the employee contribution demanded of them was too large a part of their income and they could not afford it. Employee contributions to health insurance act as a regressive tax in that the premiums represent a larger share of income for low-wage workers, and required employee contributions increase when other family members are included on the plan. For mothers who cannot afford their own health insurance, the cost of the contribution they must make for coverage of their children is almost always prohibitive. Only two of our ethnographic mothers were able to insure their entire household through employment-based plans even for short periods of time.

Co-payments and deductibles were another aspect of most employer-assisted health care plans that presented major barriers to low-income mothers. Even in those rare situations in which mothers could obtain private health insurance, they often found themselves rationing their own use of health care services because of the co-payments and the deductibles that were required. Unfortunately, neither Medicaid nor private insurance cover all medical expenses. The mothers in our study were often left with sizable expenditures even when they had health care coverage, as we learned from their stories concerning difficulties obtaining dental or eye care and of their inability to pay for all of the over-the-counter and prescription drugs and other materials recommended or prescribed by their physicians.

A Growing Problem for Working Families

We end this chapter by noting that although our study focused on the health insurance difficulties of the poor, the crisis in health care coverage is no longer confined to the bottom of the income distribution. Increasingly, instability in health care coverage, like instability in employment, is moving up the job hierarchy and affecting more working and middle-class families. If there is any hope for a change in the system, it arises from the fact that the poor are no longer the only victims. President Johnson's War on Poverty was in most respects a historical fluke, and we are unlikely to see major political initiatives to improve the lot of the poor in the near future. High rates of medical inflation and the growing vulnerability of the middle class, however, could serve as a major engine for change in the system as a whole. As we noted earlier, the major cause of bankruptcy in America today is crushing medical debt (Jacoby, Sullivan, and Warren 2000; Jacoby, Sullivan, and Warren 2001; Sullivan, Warren, and Westbrook 2000). As employers drop expensive health insurance plans or shift a larger portion of the cost of health insurance to employees, as more middle-class workers find themselves redefined as independent contractors or contingent workers, and as retirees find that the promises of lifelong health care that were made to them during their working lives are not honored, more middle-class Americans will experience the health care financing uncertainties that have historically plagued the poor. Our families then are the canaries in the mine that signal that we may all soon have something serious to worry about.

The working poor have never enjoyed true job security, and in many ways they have served as the bellwether for a new trend toward contingent and contract employment in which there is no long-term employer/employee contract or a strong sense of mutual loyalty and responsibility. The fact that the post–World War II benefit package, which included full family coverage for unionized and blue-collar workers, is eroding in value may serve as the motivation for more basic structural reform of the health care financing system. Many employers are beginning to fill some positions by contracting with secondary agencies or using temporary workers (Barker and Christensen 1998). Although many workers prefer the flexibility of such contingent employment and some contingent jobs pay relatively high wages, some of these new jobs share many of the characteristics of the jobs in which the mothers in the ethnography worked on and off. The essence of this new contingent arrangement is that the worker is not a true employee of the firm for which she works on a short-term basis. Unlike permanent employees, they are not entitled to any benefits the employer may offer, nor do they have any long-term job security.

Globalization and market uncertainty create the need for a highly flexible labor force that allows firms to react quickly to changing situations. Contingent employment, outsourcing, and just-in-time inventorying create employment environments in which the tie between employer and employee becomes looser and less paternalistic. Although certain high-productivity workers must be kept on the payroll even in slow times to ensure that they will be available in good times, production line workers, office staff, and maintenance workers are only needed on a contingent basis. Increasingly, rather than hiring one's own staff to fill maintenance, administrative, or production slots, the services these employees provide are purchased from some third party or independent contractor. By contracting out, the firm is no longer responsible for providing benefits.

In the end, our analysis of the survey data and a close examination of our ethnographic data made it clear that the employment–health insurance nexus that has served the middle class so well does not exist for those at the economic margin. Low-wage jobs are defined by sectors of the economy in which profit margins are low and in which employers face stiff competition that forces them to keep wages as low as possible. For workers in this part of the service sector, upward mobility, self-sufficiency, and adequate health care coverage remain elusive goals. Although they would have clearly preferred employer-sponsored health insurance over public coverage, our ethnographic families needed the income more than the coverage, or rather they needed both but simply could not make the income sacrifice. The situation of these families clearly revealed the inherent dilemma of an employment-based health coverage system in which jobs that pay low wages also provide no or only prohibitively expensive benefits.

In closing, we must reiterate that in discussions of poverty and the lack of health insurance race and ethnicity are unavoidable topics. One's position in the labor market and one's risk of poverty are influenced by race and ethnicity as well as by one's immigration status (Lee and Angel 2002). Massachusetts, Illinois, and Texas are among the eight states with the largest minority and noncitizen populations, groups that are disproportionately poor and politically powerless. Approximately 17 percent of noncitizens in Massachusetts and Illinois and 34 percent in Texas live in poverty (Zimmerman and Tumlin 1999). Even legal immigrants are ineligible for most public programs for a period of five years after they arrive. States differ in the services they provide to immigrants. Texas has one of the least generous insurance programs for immigrant parents and children in the nation (Capps 2001). In contrast, Massachusetts provides generous health coverage in addition to other social services for immigrants and is among the states with the highest rate of health care coverage for immigrant children in the nation (Tumlin, Zimmermann, and Ost 1999). Illinois falls somewhere between the two (Zimmerman and Tumlin 1999).

Although all the families in our ethnographic sample were selected to be potentially eligible for welfare and therefore were legal residents, Mexican-origin families occasionally talked about the impact of attitudes toward immigration and the enforcement of immigration laws on their own experiences. We quickly came to understand that immigration and citizenship were part of a complex group identity that affected individuals' experience of their minority status and that fed into their experience of powerlessness in the face of complex welfare bureaucracies. In Chapter 6, we examine how race and ethnicity influence one's experience of poverty and powerlessness and how one's identity is determined by one's interaction with the welfare system and the larger bureaucracy.

6

Confronting the System

Minority Group Identity and Powerlessness

The plight of low-income families like those in our study remains invisible and often incomprehensible to most middle-class white Americans. The poor, and particularly the minority poor, live in their own sections of town that most outsiders neither visit nor understand particularly well. What the average citizen knows about the poor is what he or she sees and hears on the evening news, gathers from the Internet, or reads in newspapers and magazines. Much of that information is negative and focuses on crime, family disruption, welfare dependence, and any number of other social pathologies. The fact that the waitresses, the busboys, the nurse's assistants, and the other service personnel that one encounters on a daily basis are so often black or speak Spanish among themselves only hints at the complex world that exists apart from America's richer neighborhoods and shopping areas. Although these low-wage workers are crucial to maintaining the high quality of life Americans enjoy, at the end of the day they return to their own neighborhoods and have little to do with the people they serve. They receive little thanks or appreciation for their efforts, and they receive even less money. They remain apart and outside the mainstream of middle-class American life.

The fact that poverty is concentrated in specific neighborhoods and among families of color continues to have serious implications for the residents of those neighborhoods, as well as for the public support of social service programs and general perceptions of welfare (Gilens 1999; Kain and Quigley 1972; Quadagno 1988; Wilson 1987). As we

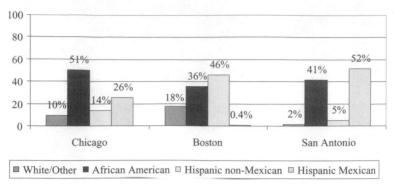

FIGURE 6.1. Race and ethnicity of primary caregiver by city

noted in Chapter 1, any study of poverty almost by definition becomes a study of race and Hispanic ethnicity. Random sampling in any of America's poor neighborhoods invariably produces samples that are largely black or Hispanic, and because we focused on low-income families, the Three City Study inevitably became a study of African Americans and Latinos. Given the centrality of the issue of race and ethnicity to economic well-being and health, we could not fail to address the issue directly.

The Racial and Ethnic Composition of the Three Cities

As middle-class Americans have abandoned the city and migrated to the suburbs, many inner-city areas, and especially the poorest neighborhoods, have become communities of color. Figure 6.1 shows that in all three of our study cities the survey samples were predominantly black and Latino. San Antonio has no predominantly poor white neighborhoods, and because our study design required that we sample in neighborhoods with concentrated poverty, our sample from there is almost completely Hispanic and African American. This concentration of poverty and minorities in specific neighborhoods was clearly a major motivation for our study, but it was not the only motivation. In addition to the fact that the poor are disproportionately minority, our focus on race and Hispanic ethnicity was motivated by the fact that, as we noted in Chapter 1, the social welfare state in the United States has been shaped by our history of race relations and the exclusion of certain groups from full civic and economic involvement. This exclusion was at one time deliberate, justified in law, and accepted convention, but more recently it has resulted from serious economic disadvantage. The Social Security Act, for example, initially excluded agricultural and domestic workers at the insistence of southern Democrats. The effect was to keep the majority of black and brown Americans from participating in the program (Davies and Derthick 1997; Hacker 2002; Lieberman 1998; Quadagno 1988; Quadagno 2005; Weir, Orloff, and Skocpol 1988). Literacy tests, poll taxes, residency requirements, and many other barriers to complete enfranchisement kept minority Americans from voting and fully participating in the political life of the nation until the passage of the Civil Rights Act of 1964 and the Voting Rights Bill of 1965 (Goodwin 1991; U.S. Department of Justice 2005).

Even with the elimination of discriminatory legal handicaps, however, other factors continue to impede the economic and social incorporation of many blacks and Hispanics. As we have seen in our previous case studies, and as we document in this chapter, economic and residential exclusion and segregation are the core components of a system of structural disadvantage that places African Americans and Hispanics at a serious disadvantage in the labor force and at a highly elevated risk of poverty and poor health. Clearly, much progress has been made in the economic and social incorporation of minority Americans, yet as we show in this chapter, the process is far from complete. This incomplete incorporation is reflected in the existence of the barrios and ghettos that occupy large areas of our major cities. The residential segregation of blacks and Latinos in socially isolated neighborhoods that offer few local job opportunities and that are located long distances from such opportunities limits the employment options of a large fraction of minority individuals. As we show, ghettoized communities have few collective or institutional resources, and survival in them requires networks of mutual support. Unfortunately, although such networks are crucial for survival, the need to share one's limited resources with others limits one's ability to save and undermines the ability of individuals and families to get ahead.

Residential segregation has several causes. Historically, it has been a normal aspect of the incorporation of immigrant groups. Yet for some African Americans and Latinos residential segregation has not been a passing phase in a process of full social and economic incorporation (Massey and Denton 1993; Portes and Bach 1985; Portes and

Rumbaut 1997). For the African American population, it is the result of a long history of slavery, racism, and discrimination. Certain Hispanic groups, including Puerto Ricans and Dominicans, are of mixed race and are subject to the same sorts of discrimination. For the Mexican-origin population, a unique set of institutional factors has kept many members of that group from moving into the social and economic mainstream. Even during the post–World War II period of prosperity, the Mexican American population lagged behind non-Hispanic whites in capital accumulation (Grebler, Moore, and Guzman 1970). The unique nature of labor markets in the Southwest and the heavy concentration of Mexican-origin workers in agricultural and manual labor are among the factors that have kept them from achieving economic parity with the majority (Capps, Fix, and Passel 2003; Kazis and Miller 2001; Taylor, Martin, and Fix 1997).

For Hispanics, of course, an important aspect of group identity is language. Although most long-term residents speak fluent English, a substantial fraction of the Mexican-origin population, including recent immigrants, are not fluent in English. A lack of English proficiency and the inability to easily navigate large and confusing bureaucracies present very practical problems related to understanding the requirements for social program participation and being able to fill out forms. The inability to communicate fluently in English or speaking with a strong accent also labels one as an outsider. Language and cultural differences translate directly into differences in social standing.

The asymmetries of power, authority, and social standing that are an inevitable part of interactions between clients and impersonal bureaucracies take their toll in terms of one's ability to acquire the services for which one applies and in terms of lowered self-esteem and damage to one's sense of personal efficacy. Many of the women we interviewed spoke repeatedly of the humiliation involved in conversations at the welfare office in which they were accused of lying, spoken to in a condescending manner, or otherwise demeaned.

Vulnerability, Group Membership, and Health

In this chapter, we deal with the analytically difficult issues of race and Hispanic ethnicity, minority-group status, and social exclusion in order to illustrate how minority-group membership relates to increased vulnerability and difficulties in obtaining social services, including those related to health care. We explore the extent to which those experiences related to race, ethnicity, and powerlessness form part of a cycle of poverty in which the inability to exert control over bureaucratic processes, in combination with low levels of community resources and burdensome family responsibilities, reinforces one's inferior social status and undermines one's ability to engage in instrumental action. As Oscar Lewis attempted to elaborate decades ago, poverty has negative consequences for all aspects of subjective experience as the result of a lack of objective control over the circumstances of one's life (Lewis 1959; 1966). Lewis was severely criticized for supposedly attributing an individual's failure to move ahead in life to the belief and behavioral systems into which the poor are socialized rather than to the social structures that impede their social and economic mobility.

Given the all too common practice of blaming the poor for their own plight, we would not want to reinforce conceptions of a culture of poverty that fail to adequately account for the structural factors related to the educational system, the labor market, and the social welfare system that impede the efforts of minority Americans to advance socially and economically. Although individual behaviors clearly influence one's level of social mobility, it is clear that one's possibilities for mobility are greatly conditioned by opportunities that are not distributed randomly but are affected greatly by group membership. Nonetheless, our observations have been that individuals who grow up in poverty, especially if they are members of stigmatized groups, spend much of their lives embedded in a symbolic world in which those symbols clearly differentiate the rich from the poor and the powerful from the weak and at every turn remind one that he or she is not one of the rich or powerful. When the color distinctions are as stark as they continue to be in the United States, the impact of race and ethnicity on the experience of poverty cannot be ignored, even if in a post–civil rights era the nation has lost interest in the topic. In what follows, we draw primarily upon our ethnographic data to illustrate the overt and more subtle ways in which the symbolic aspects of poverty, as they are confounded by those of race and Hispanic ethnicity, give rise to potentially serious demoralization that in conjunction with real structural barriers to personal and group advancement seriously undermine individuals' and families' life chances.

Fifty years of statistical analysis clearly document the economic and social disadvantages suffered by blacks and Hispanics. Yet the disadvantages they suffer are not confined solely to economics or social status. Because of the increased risk of poverty of both groups, they face an elevated risk of poor health from those diseases associated with poverty. As we documented in earlier chapters, the poor suffer more morbidity and die at higher rates than the middle class because they are exposed to more health risks and receive poorer-quality health care. In addition, they also suffer from another health risk that is as serious as any other – discrimination. A growing body of evidence reveals that both the overt and more subtle forms of discrimination that minority Americans experience daily undermine their physical and mental health (Finch, Kolody, and Vega 2000; Jackson et al. 1996; Kessler, Mickelson, and Williams 1999; Kreiger, Sidney, and Coakley 1999; Sellers and Shelton 2003). The data clearly indicate that there is something about minority-group membership, above and beyond its association with low socioeconomic status, that undermines health and well-being. Our conversations with poor women who had to seek assistance led us to the conclusion that like perceived discrimination, the frequent demeaning experiences that the poor must endure in their daily lives and in their interactions with the bureaucracy undermine their general well-being.

The case studies that follow illustrate how ethnicity and minority-group status influenced aspects of identity among our respondents and how their subjective experience of their social and economic inferiority was related to their inability to control important aspects of their lives. Although we focus on health and health care generally, issues of control, or the lack of it, pervaded all aspects of their lives, and our conversations concerning health and interactions with the bureaucracy touched upon many other issues in which the lack of power or control over events was relevant. Much of this lack of control resulted from invidious social comparisons with those who were better-off and of a different race or ethnicity, but also from the hugely asymmetrical relationship between low-income powerless recipients of services and incomprehensible and what at times seemed like irrational bureaucracies. Gaining insight into whether and how our respondents perceived that their race or ethnicity related to their poverty was not easy, largely because, as we have noted, race and ethnicity are factors that affect all aspects of life and share the taken-for-granted quality of many aspects of identity even for non-Hispanic whites who are the beneficiaries of racial inequalities (McIntosh 1990).

Illuminating the role that race and ethnicity played in the lives of the women in our study was made more difficult by the fact that racial and ethnic identities are complex psychological constructions that are influenced by many individual and social factors (Phinney 1990). Different individuals hold different conceptions of themselves as members of specific groups, and simple survey questions related to one's racial- and ethnic-group members that limit one's choice of responses no doubt greatly simplify what are in reality complex social and cultural constructions. With few exceptions, our respondents talked more about their problems with jobs and their problems with the welfare bureaucracy than about issues specific to their race or ethnicity, even when it was clear that race and ethnicity mattered and were a major reason for their vulnerability. Being poor and Mexican may well place one in the barrio or in public housing, but what our respondents talked to us about were the problems of the barrio or their housing. They told us about their daily struggles, the difficulties they encountered in setting and achieving goals for themselves and their children, and the stigma of being at the bottom in an affluent society. They were conscious of being poor and of living at the margin, but they did not frame, or at least they did not for the most part articulate, their problems in terms of race or ethnicity.

What we found was that the vulnerabilities associated with being African American or Mexican as they related to access to education, access to jobs, and dependence on at least some parts of the welfare system were described and expressed through the experience and language of powerlessness in the face of bureaucracies established and run by unknown powers. Although some families accepted, or at least appeared to have become resigned to, the vagaries of the welfare system, others were engaged in a continuous struggle with it, and the fact that they were not powerful clients came across in our conversations. What was clear was that the identity that they had to assume as welfare recipients was confounded in complex and sometimes subtle ways with their racial and ethnic group identities, often in ways that made a positive attitude and effective instrumental action all the more difficult.

We might usefully summarize our understanding of the experience of race and Hispanic ethnicity and their consequences by noting that ethnic or racial identity and group membership related most clearly to our families' experiences in three ways that most of our respondents talked about in some detail. These had to do with inadequate housing and disorganized neighborhoods, difficulties in obtaining education and training, and the fact that poverty forced poor families to depend on one another. All three of these problem domains are influenced by the extent of the racial and ethnically based segregation of urban communities generally. It is no accident that members of ethnic and racial minorities tend to live in highly segregated poor communities and that segregation itself, whether the result of formal policies as in the past or the result of economic inequality that seriously restricts residential mobility among the poor today, continues to have serious negative personal and social consequences. Our study families directly experienced the reality of functionally segregated neighborhoods, schools, and labor markets. Even well after the era of Jim Crow and the restrictive covenants and redlining that forced blacks and Latinos into ghettos and barrios, the economic reality of their lives means that they live with other low-income families of color. As a result of their geographic concentration, their children attend the same schools, and because of their own limited educations and opportunities, they work in the same sorts of jobs.

The Barrio and the Intergenerational Transmission of Poverty

For low-income minority families, a lack of education and job skills represents a major barrier to mobility, and our sample provided few exceptions. Most of our respondents had grown up in the same sort of economically depressed ethnic or racial enclaves in which they currently lived. For these individuals, poverty had been transmitted intergenerationally. By and large, our respondents had gone to inferior strife-ridden ghetto or barrio schools and had low levels of education. They had limited access to high-level job training and preparation programs and often had early histories of poor health. Such early life handicaps had a lifelong impact on their opportunities, and they were well aware of that fact. The limited human capital that was the result of these early handicaps continued to interact with the powerlessness of their social location to perpetuate their economic vulnerability.

Finally, the fact that they had few personal resources was compounded by the limited neighborhood and community resources available in most poor communities, and it meant that they were forced to spend their energy and their limited material resources on caring for others as well as for themselves. The individual social mobility that has characterized most middle-class families since the early 1990s requires that one save to improve the material aspects of one's life and to provide one's children with educational and other opportunities. Among the poor, the needs of family members, relatives, and neighbors draw upon a family's limited resources and make such savings almost impossible. Our data, like those of other researchers, revealed the degree of the burden that poor families must assume for other relatives and even for nonrelatives. Survival in low-income resource-poor neighborhoods requires a mutual interdependence, and many women find themselves responsible not only for their own families but for others in extended networks of kin and close friends (Berick 1995; Hays 2003; Rank 1994; Stack 1997).

Demoralization

As we collected data on family structure, marital and romantic histories, child care, health care, and much more concerning these families' lives, we could not help but ask ourselves how anyone could deal with the constant instability and disappointment that so many experienced on an almost daily basis. Psychiatric epidemiologists have developed the concept of "demoralization" to characterize the nonspecific psychological distress that people experience in certain situations that they cannot control (Dohrenwend et al. 1980; Gutkovich et al. 1999; Rickelman 2002). The concept struck us as uniquely appropriate to the settings in which we worked. Rather than conveying a narrow clinical meaning, the concept of demoralization conveys a more general sense of hopelessness and helplessness, indeed of powerlessness, in multiple domains of life that has its origin in the objective circumstances of individuals' and groups' lives. Our African American and Latino families seemed particularly vulnerable to demoralization given their poverty and powerlessness. Why, we asked ourselves, don't people in these situations just give up? What we observed was that most struggle on because they have no choice and, most importantly perhaps, because they have children for whom they feel a deep parental responsibility. A few, as we will see, even seemed to develop some sense of control, but many lives were clearly blighted by the demoralization that is an inevitable result of a stigmatized identity and the inability to control important aspects of life. We came to realize that the bureaucracies with which the poor must interact in order to survive are structured in such a way as to increase rather than reduce the number of obstacles they must overcome and to increase their sense of powerlessness and their demoralization.

Despite the fact that these families had few resources and had to deal with often intransigent bureaucracies, they also developed effective survival strategies with which to compensate for their absence of economic or social influence. As we have seen in previous chapters, these strategies were centered on a constant effort to gain some control over their lives, particularly in terms of the welfare of their children. When it was successful, their perseverance paid off in terms of the enhanced cohesion and strength of their families, their success in providing for their children, and their ability to negotiate and successfully employ a complex organizational environment. They learned to combine the services of formal governmental institutions to obtain TANF, food stamps, and Medicaid to obtain the basics of daily life, and more informal nongovernmental organizations, such as churches, food pantries, and other charitable organizations, for more episodic assistance.

It is clearly important for us to recognize the effectiveness that many families displayed in these efforts and also to recognize the real courage of their efforts. However, they found themselves in situations in which a large fraction, if not the majority, of their time and energy had to be devoted to obtaining the real basics of daily life. Unfortunately, their attempts to keep their households intact and their children healthy and supervised were not always successful. Most families in our sample were minorities, and most were attempting these challenging tasks in neighborhoods beset with crime, drugs, and general social disorganization, problems that interact with race and ethnicity to create low levels of economic opportunity (Wilson 1987). The fact that so much of their time had to be devoted to basics meant that little was left to devote to educational programs or efforts to enhance job skills. The result was often a trap in which the lack of opportunity for social mobility or economic advancement fed back into a general community sense of demoralization.

In our interviews, we heard from unique individuals with different temperaments and different capacities for dealing with the difficulties in their lives. Like the majority of our sample, however, they share the reality of their minority-group status. As we have noted, few of our respondents overtly attributed their circumstances to the fact of their race or ethnicity. Of course, we did not probe directly for their conceptions of how their race or ethnicity affected their lives. Our conversations were more general and focused on daily routines, interactions with the welfare bureaucracy, and daily hassles. In this context, few of our respondents talked much about race or ethnicity at all. Some even rejected a racial or ethnic attribution for their problems. As one young African American mother of two boys told us, "I consider myself a person. I am a human being. I don't consider myself no African American or black or nothing like that. I am a person, period." This young mother told us that she did not talk to her children about race because she did not want them to focus on their color.

Despite the fact that this young mother did not want to talk about race, like most of our other study families she and her sons lived in a world defined by their racial and ethnic identity and largely distinct and separate from that of middle-class white America. What we found was that rather than defining themselves as racial or ethnic group members, the consciousness of minority-group status was confounded with aspects of social class powerlessness, and our respondents articulated the reality of their lives more in terms of powerlessness in the face of their poverty and the impenetrable and confusing bureaucracies that they were forced to rely on rather than overtly in terms of race or ethnicity. Although the stories we have already presented clearly demonstrate the powerlessness and lack of control that our families experienced, in this chapter we present several more cases to focus a clearer light on how race and Hispanic ethnicity are experienced in real-life contexts.

Yvonne

We met Yvonne, a thirty-year-old Mexican American mother of five, shortly after she had moved into The Courts. The housing project consisted almost entirely of Mexican-origin families. Yvonne's friends and neighbors were all Mexican, and the neighborhood truly felt like a Mexican community. Like much project housing, the building in which Yvonne and her family lived was not in good shape. To get to the apartment, the interviewer had to climb a damp, grimy, and littered stairwell. The Courts dominated the neighborhood, and because it was spread out over a large area it created a considerable zone with few businesses and limited public transportation.

Our first interview took place on a hot summer day, and the window air-conditioning unit in one room could not keep the apartment cool. In addition to Yvonne, the family consisted of a daughter age three, four sons, ages five, seven, eleven, and fourteen, and Yvonne's new partner, who was not the father of any of her five children. His children were also living in the apartment, as was one of Yvonne's nieces and her baby. Occasionally a nephew who split his time between Yvonne's apartment and his mother's house also stayed with the family. With so many people, the apartment was crowded and Yvonne was challenged to keep order and to keep up basic maintenance. Such overcrowding is a major problem for many poor families, especially for Mexican Americans, who have high fertility rates and large extended families. Lacking resources or a safety net, the poor must look to relatives and friends as a last resort in dealing with problems. The traditional stereotype of large extended Mexican families living in crowded dwelling units by choice may, in fact, represent less a cultural preference and more simple necessity. Yvonne's acceptance of so many relatives represents her contribution to a mutual support network on which she may at some point be forced to rely.

Although we deliberately oversampled families with a disabled member, many of the families in our study who were not members of this oversample were caring for someone with a physical or mental handicap. The fact that blacks and Hispanics are at elevated risk of poverty and its health risks means that many families must care for family members with serious disabilities, and they must do so in difficult and trying circumstances. Yvonne's oldest son was disabled and mentally retarded. He attended a special eighth-grade program at the local public school because he read at the first-grade level. There were few other programs available to him, and caring for him took a great deal of time because he needed assistance in dressing and other daily activities. Because of his severe disability the boy was eligible for supplemental security income (SSI), and the family received a monthly stipend. Supplemental security income automatically qualifies one for Medicaid, so at least this son was continuously covered for his medical care.

Yvonne had always lived in the barrio, and she grew up in a large, strife-ridden family. Her mother and father had four daughters together, but they separated while Yvonne was still a baby, and each had more children with other partners. With so many children, they could do little for any of them, and their lives embodied the stereotype of uncontrolled fertility that is so often attributed to minority individuals. Yvonne's mother had been diagnosed with AIDS and lived with Yvonne's sister. When we met Yvonne, she was dealing with the first of several health problems of which we became aware. Like most of our sample, she had no health insurance or any hope of ever acquiring employer coverage. She had been on and off Medicaid over the previous several years, but Medicaid did not always cover her prescribed treatments.

At the time of our interviews, Yvonne was suffering from rash-like bumps that itched unbearably and that were eventually diagnosed as flea bites to which she was allergic. She also suffered from the long-term effects of a childhood spinal injury that made it hard for her to meet the demands of her grocery store job and that required narcotic drugs to manage the pain. A few months after we met her, she and four of the five children developed a strep infection, and Yvonne lost several days of work because she had to remain home to recuperate and care for the children. Like many of the mothers we met, Yvonne's residence in a segregated and resource-poor neighborhood with only limited access to transportation seriously restricted her employment opportunities. With few other employment opportunities, Yvonne, like many other mothers in such segregated neighborhoods, often took jobs in the informal economy. Both African American and Mexican American mothers often worked at informal jobs where they were paid in cash and had no benefits and no security.

Over the eighteen-month period that we worked with Yvonne, she held four different jobs. None offered much income or stability, and none helped Yvonne feel good about herself. The first job was at a cafe, where she was paid cash by her employer, who did not pay Social

Security taxes for his employees. The long-term consequences of such informal work are, of course, serious. Not only does one not earn enough to save for the future, but also because one pays no Social Security taxes one can easily fail to make the required ten years of contributions necessary to receive benefits. Even if Yvonne were to qualify, however, the small size of her contributions would entitle her only to the lowest stipend. Although we did not include undocumented workers in our study, those individuals are even more vulnerable to employer exploitation than citizens. Even for citizens, however, the fact of being Mexican with little education and few resources increases one's vulnerability in the job market.

The informal nature of her job caused other problems for Yvonne. At the time, she was in a special housing program that required that she find work within three months. Because the job was informal, the employer would not write a letter to the housing authority documenting her employment, so the job could not meet the requirements of the housing program. Faced with the possibility of eviction, Yvonne quit the cafe job and took a job in food service, but she quit that second job within the week. That job began at 6 A.M., and there was no public transportation running at that hour. Taking a cab was too expensive given the job's low wages, so Yvonne took a third job. For one month, she worked as a seasonal cashier at a local store, but that temporary position soon ended. Within a month, she took a fourth position, this time at the local grocery store. That job was typical of many of the service-sector jobs our respondents found. In most restaurants, construction sites, hotels and motels, and other service industries in the Southwest and increasingly in other parts of the country, cleaning and service staffs are largely Mexican and Mexican American, as are almost all of those working as agricultural labor (Capps, Fix, and Passel 2003; Kazis and Miller 2001; Taylor, Martin, and Fix 1997). None of Yvonne's four jobs provided enough work or income for her to support her family.

Throughout this period of the study, the family was on TANF, although the amounts varied considerably, adding to the ongoing uncertainty of Yvonne's life. Yvonne was penalized during one of her job searches because she had not been able to submit the fifteen job applications in one week that were required. In a limited local formal economy, typical of many depressed ethnic-minority communities, it is difficult to locate potential employers, and the travel time to apply outside the community makes it difficult to submit numerous applications in a week. On another occasion, Yvonne was penalized because one of her children was late for a required physical examination. She told us that she had made the appointment, but her doctor was backed up for several months and could not see the child within the TANF-imposed deadline.

Yvonne was still trying to continue her education and had only two exams left to earn her GED. It was clear that one of her defenses against demoralization was a strong belief in education and the hope that with education her children would escape poverty. As she told us,

I stress education to kids so much, and I would love, I swear, to get a college education for myself to do what I've always wanted to do, to get my college education, get my career. . . . I always tell people it wasn't that I was stupid and I couldn't go to school. . . . I mean most of the time I didn't even go to school because my mother never came home and I had to stay home with the other little kids at home, you know! I flunked the seventh grade.

When the study ended, Yvonne and her family were struggling to get by, but it was clear to us that their precarious situation would probably never improve because of the interaction of so many negative factors. The family was still trapped in a resource-poor neighborhood with few local job opportunities. Yvonne continued to juggle multiple and demanding responsibilities for her immediate family and for a much larger network, responsibilities that quickly drained off whatever resources she was able to accumulate. Despite it all, however, she was continuing her attempts to educate herself and her children. We left the family with the hope that Yvonne will see her children succeed and her own efforts on their behalf rewarded. It was clear, however, that the fact that she was Mexican placed her at a distinct disadvantage in terms of access to the means of achieving that success.

Sonia

Although Sonia faced a series of responsibilities for her family network, she stood out because, unlike so many of the families we talked to, she felt empowered even as she seemed to face daunting obstacles. An African American grandmother with custody of her two grandsons, ages fourteen and sixteen, Sonia took her responsibilities as their guardian very seriously and was heavily involved in the boys' care and upbringing. The exact circumstances that led to Sonia's taking formal custody of her grandsons remained unclear, and we did not push her for more specifics than she was willing to volunteer; however, we did find out that the custody arrangement was the result of her daughter's use of drugs. Sonia, however, was unusual. She definitely saw herself as her grandsons' primary socializing agent and protector, and she fought to make sure they had access to various programs, including health care. Unlike most of the mothers we met, Sonia expressed a sense of competence in dealing with the welfare bureaucracy. She did not feel or express herself as though she were a helpless pawn in the system. Quite the contrary, she felt empowered to demand what she felt her grandsons deserved and felt competent to extract it from the systems with which she dealt.

One could hardly help but be impressed by Sonia's strength of character and her determination. She attributed her willingness and ability to engage the system to the influence of the politically active family in which she grew up. She told us that she also learned a great deal from the legal aid services in another city, which she had used to educate herself about the law. She had attended information sessions at legal aid services and also visited legislative offices where she could learn "what her rights were." Whether her attitude was the result of an innate positive temperament or her family's influence, Sonia stood out as unusual in her sense of competency to get what she needed from the bureaucracies she faced.

Like many of the mothers in our study, Sonia had been repeatedly denied welfare and associated services for her grandsons. However, as a woman who would not take "no" for an answer when she knew she was in the right, she vigorously set herself to the task of reversing the denials and had been successful in almost all cases. When we met her, the two boys were on SSI and Medicaid. A successful application for SSI almost always requires a lawyer because establishing eligibility is a complex process. Sonia's older grandson had both hearing and learning disabilities, and the younger boy had sickle-cell anemia and other associated health problems. Sonia explained to us that one of the boys was dropped from SSI for a period of time, but Sonia appealed the termination and attended a hearing where she served as her own advocate. With the support of the boy's doctor, she regained the SSI, and her two grandsons have been continuously covered by SSI and Medicaid since then.

Sonia was creative and energetic in her efforts to keep the welfare, food stamps, and Medicaid she and her grandsons needed. She described with gusto her altercations with various welfare offices, occasionally drawing on a little poetic license. During one particularly contentious altercation with the welfare office, she wrote to her congressional representative, who intervened on Sonia's behalf. Sonia attributed the rapid and positive response by the welfare office to her willingness to take drastic action when necessary. It probably would not have occurred to many other women in her situation to bring political pressure to bear on the welfare bureaucracy. On another occasion, the state office told her that her documentation had been lost. Over their objections, she insisted on personally taking the paperwork to the comptroller's office in order to receive her check as soon as possible.

Sonia explained that "if you want your money you have to be persistent." During one episode of illness, her grandson was hospitalized off and on for over three months. The total bill was very large, but it was supposed to be paid by Medicaid. For some reason, however, the charges were denied. Again Sonia did not simply accept the judgment and worked with legal aid for two years to clear the debt. The basic principle that she lived by was that dealing successfully with the welfare office took a great deal of time, work, and knowledge. She believed that if she did not fight for her rights and those of her family, she would become a victim, and she was not willing to do so.

Sonia's efforts, or at least her account of them, reflected an effective use of the poverty programs on which poor families depend rather than movement toward real self-sufficiency. Ill herself, and living in a resource-poor neighborhood, Sonia had little access to jobs and little probability of ever obtaining the kind of job that would support her complex household and provide the full range of medical care all of its members needed. She, like most of the other families in the study, found herself embedded in an extended family network that placed additional demands on her time, energy, and material resources. On a daily basis, she shouldered burdens that required the complex support of multiple agencies. Again, the combination of limitations on Sonia's own opportunities, the resource-poor community in which she lived, and her responsibilities for children with multiple needs made her dependent on welfare services and left little room for change in her overall economic status. As with Yvonne, Sonia rarely referred to race in her discussions of her own situation; however, she talked often about the welfare bureaucracies, the neighborhood resources or lack thereof, and the responsibilities she faced. Yet, in Sonia's case, it was clear that the situation in which the family found itself was clearly influenced by race.

Claudia

Few women in Sonia's situation had her knowledge, strength, and stamina. Unfortunately, for most poor mothers, the battle for benefits was often a losing one, and many simply went without the basic benefits for which they supposedly qualified on the basis of need or for which they did not qualify because even their rather meager earnings were too high for them to be eligible. At the other end of the spectrum were mothers like Claudia, who found it difficult either to locate or keep a job because of the demands of maintaining welfare support. Claudia, a young African American mother of two sons, ages four and five, was receiving Medicaid for herself and the two boys when she joined the study. She struggled continuously to keep the coverage. When we met her, she had only one year of TANF eligibility left. Among Claudia's struggles was an ongoing effort to get child support from the father of her older son. She had been receiving TANF since the older boy was born and had been trying unsuccessfully to get child support from his father since then. The office where she applied for assistance in getting child support was in the same building in which she applied and recertified her eligibility for TANF. She not only was required by the welfare system to seek child support from the father but also felt it was the father's responsibility and that he was shirking it. Unfortunately, like so many absent fathers who have never known their children, he evidently felt little obligation to his son. Keeping track of the father's whereabouts was difficult because he changed jobs as often as every week or two and it was hard for Claudia to locate him and to try to get him to pay. Claudia felt that obtaining the child support was all up to her because she got little help from the welfare system in arranging the child support that they required.

Because she wished to move to a nicer apartment, Claudia had applied for subsidized housing, and she had been on that waiting list for at least three years. Once she finally received the voucher that she could use to pay the rent, she had a short period of time within which to find a landlord who would accept it. Although she might have been able to find an apartment, she had no savings, and the housing authority would not assist her with the initial deposit. Because she could not come up with the deposit, the window of opportunity closed before she was able to locate an apartment for which she could qualify with only the minimal deposit she could make. As a result, she again went to the end of the waiting list. It was hard to imagine that when she got to the head of the list again Claudia would be in any better situation to take advantage of it.

Claudia's failure to move the family to a nicer apartment was typical of her inability to use the welfare system to her advantage, and experiences like these were clearly demoralizing. Without child support and with the two young children, she had Medicaid, TANF, and food stamps, at least for the moment. However, because of the time limits imposed on TANF, she would lose cash assistance within a year, and she had no clear plan as to what she would do when that occurred. The future seemed bleak because, as was the case for most of the families we studied, finding a steady job with benefits was an unrealistic goal. When we were last in contact with Claudia, she was starting to look for work, but it was unclear whether she would be able to find appropriate child care, or whether she would receive assistance in paying for it. Even with a child care subsidy, she would have to locate the child care herself, and she was uncertain that she would be able to do so. Claudia also did not know how she would maintain health insurance for herself once she was off welfare. Claudia's situation was much more typical of our families than was Sonia's. She tried but was frequently unsuccessful in combining her ongoing search for a job, the requirements of the welfare system, and the other responsibilities of her life.

Of course, because we were relying on accounts of past events from our respondents themselves, we cannot confirm the accuracy of their information. All of the narratives contained inconsistencies that we were unable to reconcile and that, as we mentioned in Chapter 1, probably reflect the vagaries of human memory as well as the complexity of the situations that the families were facing rather than any desire to deceive. Whether Sonia was actually as effective in dealing with the welfare bureaucracy as she claimed to be we cannot verify. Nonetheless, the important point for our purposes is that Sonia felt that she was in control of her interactions with the welfare system, whereas Yvonne and Claudia did not. Perhaps even an unrealistic sense of control serves as a buttress against the demoralization that one might so easily fall into. Realistically, a poor family's control over important aspects of its life is limited. What Yvonne, Sonia, and Claudia shared in common, was that they were minority Americans. Each lived in an impoverished neighborhood, and each faced multiple heavy responsibilities with relatively few resources and few opportunities to increase their human capital and earning potential. All of these handicaps were clearly related to race and Hispanic ethnicity.

The Barrio

As these cases illustrate, one of the major mechanisms through which race and ethnicity affect life chances and health relates to the highly segregated nature of minority poor communities. Low-wage minority Americans live apart from the middle class in neighborhoods that many of our respondents characterized as having inferior schools and inadequate transportation or other public services. To many white Americans, the burden that our system of race-based social inequality imposes on individuals of color is unknown, and many clearly believe that serious inequalities have ceased to exist (McIntosh 1990). Unfortunately, serious inequalities and their negative consequences persist even today. The consequences of "ghettoization" and social exclusion are clearly detrimental for individuals and for the ghettoized group as a whole. Depressed individual earnings and limited asset accumulation translate directly into limited group assets and the deprivation-based interdependency that we noted among our study families. Residential segregation in impoverished neighborhoods with low levels of home ownership, little employment diversity, and few resources not only makes it difficult for families to save and to pass wealth on to future generations but also undermines the collective ability of a group to accumulate capital and increase their economic power (Goldscheider and Goldscheider 1991; Shapiro 2003).

Such ghettoization results from overt discrimination as well as the inability of poor families to afford more expensive housing in better neighborhoods. It also reflects public housing policy and the placement and management of the public housing developments that dominate many poor neighborhoods. As our study revealed, even outside of the projects, subsidized housing is rarely located in more affluent neighborhoods. The literature documents, and our interviews corroborate, the resulting mismatch for residents of impoverished neighborhoods between residential location and economic opportunities (Glaeser, Hanuskek, and Quigley 2004; Kain and Quigley 1972). Residential isolation in a neighborhood that is a long distance from employment opportunities when one must rely on public transportation limits a worker's job options.

The fact of residential segregation, visible in all of the neighborhoods where we interviewed, relates directly to the issue of identity. Just as they found themselves in the waiting room rather than behind the desk at the Medicaid office, our families were relegated to neighborhoods and housing for the poor where those with more resources would not choose to live. In the same way that a counter or desk reifies the social distance between the welfare applicant and the representative of the system, poor neighborhoods, with their lack of amenities and natural beauty, reify the distance between the haves and the have-nots and play into the consciousness of the latter. In the course of our study, we were reminded time and again of how pervasive the symbols of powerlessness and dependency were in the lives of the families we studied and how they contributed to a cultural environment that undermined a sense of instrumental effectiveness. It is very difficult for those who do not live with such symbols of powerlessness and the experiences that accompany them to understand what the pervasive nature of poverty can do to the human spirit and to mental and physical health.

They Look Down on Us

As the case of the bank teller we mentioned in the previous chapter shows, one's group membership is an inescapable part of one's identity. Through hard work, the teller had been promoted to a higher position as a customer service representative and transferred to a branch where she was the only Hispanic. Although it is possible that her performance in the new position required improvement, the fact that her previous performance evaluations had been good enough to earn her a promotion and the fact that her most recent evaluations were good, in addition to the nature of the criticisms she received from the supervisor at the new branch and especially the gratuitous reference to her ethnicity, make the critical evaluation suspect. The interviewer's opinion was that her command of English was very good. Once outside of their neighborhoods or their part of town, minority Americans are often made aware of their stranger status in very direct ways.

A few of our respondents did talk about their race or ethnicity as an issue in their access to public services, including medical coverage, but more of them mentioned the negative perceptions that they believed caseworkers and other program personnel had of them because of their poverty and their need to apply for welfare. Our respondents felt that, particularly in welfare offices, their social position and role as paupers became central and affected every aspect of the experience of applying for benefits as well as the likelihood that they would receive them. Our respondents only occasionally attributed difficulties in their lives to race or being Hispanic. In many domains outside of social program participation, however, it was clear to them that their poverty and lower social class were the root cause of their dilemmas. The fact that they were poor and powerless was no accident, however and in our interviews it was clear that their race and ethnicity colored how they believed they were seen and treated when they came into contact with any bureaucracy. Although some mothers reported cordial and even respectful relationships with caseworkers, many others believed that the system operated to debase and humiliate them. They interpreted the treatment they received as a continual reminder of their poverty status. One respondent explained that some caseworkers believe that clients lie. She felt that they judged everybody.

They don't respect the people. For example, if you need an application, you have to stand in line, and they ask a lot of questions before they even give you the application, and if they think you don't need it, they don't give it to you. They ask questions like, "If you have income, if you work, how have you been making it with no income?"

One Latina mother, Graciela, who lived in Chicago, confirmed that a level of suspiciousness and a lack of trust existed between clients and caseworkers, a theme we heard repeated in all three cities, and this suspiciousness was often colored by racial and ethnic group differences. By the very nature of their role, caseworkers were seen as "gatekeepers" in the application and recertification processes, as indeed they were. In the opinion of many of the respondents, if a caseworker believed that a family was either ineligible for a service or that the family really did not need the service based on the supporting material, or if the caseworker suspected that the family had other resources, he or she might well refuse to accept the application. Graciela, also like many other mothers, often felt demeaned by the nature of her interactions with welfare caseworkers because such interactions were completely asymmetrical and she was clearly powerless: "The caseworker doesn't care. She makes people wait for a long time." When Graciela attempted to apply for food stamps, her caseworker thought she made too much money to qualify or that she was at most eligible for only $45 in assistance. But as Graciela explained, even $45 "would help a lot...; it would be one month of food." So she persisted while the caseworker resisted. As she said, "The caseworker made it seem like why would you want just $45?" The caseworker never agreed to provide the forms necessary for her to apply for food stamps. Finally, when Graciela went to drop off a different application for medical coverage, she simply took one of the applications for food stamps and filled it in herself. By the time we met her, she no longer even wanted to talk to her caseworker. Whenever she could, she just mailed required documents to the welfare office and avoided interacting with caseworkers.

The issue of demeaning treatment by caseworkers and other bureaucrats came up often, and it was clear that the women felt their inferiority keenly in dealing with the system. The impacts of race and ethnicity are often subtle or indirect in that, as we have explained, they are confounded with differences in wealth, power, and organizational position. Even if one's caseworker or even if many of the caseworkers at the welfare office are of the same racial or ethnic group as oneself, the clients in the system are minority and the real power brokers and decision makers in the system are white. This racially and ethnically based gulf is palpable in its impact and colors the subjective experience of everyone involved. This is another pervasive phenomenon in the lives of the poor that is commented on only occasionally. Even when there are minority police officers on the beat in poor neighborhoods, the police department is seen as an agent of the white power structure.

The sources of humiliation and the reminder of one's inferior status pervade the welfare system and often seem to operate to undermine a person's attempts to gain self-respect. Given the fact that TANF stipends are low, particularly in Texas, most poor mothers are caught in a dilemma that arises from the fact that they have to find additional income in order to make ends meet. The cash assistance they receive is simply not enough, and most must find some additional source of money or in-kind support. (It is also clear that the income from a low-wage service-sector job is also insufficient to support a family.) However, any additional income must be reported to the welfare office and almost invariably results in the reduction of a family's TANF payment. Such a situation places poor women in the demeaning situation of having to lie about any additional income they bring in or accepting the almost impossible situation of living on welfare or a low-wage job. Again, the rules, which at times almost seem irrational, continually remind these women of their inferior and powerless positions.

One mother commented that the way they explain things at the office rather than what they tell you is "ugly." She said, "You feel low.... You say to yourself,... if I take my time to go around all day and pick up cans, I've got to report this to these people? ... If I baby-sit somebody's kid and make ten dollars, they say you have to report that." In the interactions with bureaucrats that she described, this mother, like many of the women we interviewed, was forced, on the one hand, to emphasize her own poverty and powerlessness in order to qualify for the help she could not do without and, on the other, to dissemble about the hard work and cleverness she put into strategies to make things work for her family.

Although most respondents talked in terms of how their poverty and their low levels of education were the cause of the humiliation they endured, some of the mothers in our study were more specific in talking about the impact of race on their experiences with the welfare system. In response to the question "Do some people get treated better or worse than others?" one mother answered as follows:

Yes. People that have a lighter complexion, white people, they get better treated. We as Hispanics get treated automatically badly or they talk to us rudely because they think we don't know what we're doing; we're just taking advantage and we don't want to further ourselves. So they automatically think badly and talk badly to us. They think they can walk all over us. That's why when I go I have to speak up and let them know that [even though] I'm

Hispanic and I'm on welfare, I'm trying to better myself. That doesn't give them the right...to walk all over me. Because I know what they're telling me and I know what I have to do. They think we're dumb and we don't know, but we do know. Then they won't be able to walk all over me. They know where they stand with me.

Such overt ethnic attributions were rare, but our respondents were clearly aware of how the racial concentration of the poor neighborhoods in which they lived, their group identity, and particularly the poverty that peruaded the neighborhoods in which they lived limited their opportunities and their ability to obtain education, increase their earnings, and offer a better life to their children.

Conflict and Barriers to Coalition Building

One destructive aspect of race relations in the United States is the degree to which different disadvantaged groups often find themselves in conflict with other disadvantaged groups. In San Antonio, we observed a great deal of conflict and ill will between African Americans and Mexicans as they vied for housing and other limited public resources. Sheila was one of the few non-Hispanic white women in our study. She was the mother of two children, ages three and four. Although she was not Hispanic, her husband, who was the father of her children, was Hispanic, and Sheila had lived in Hispanic neighborhoods for much of her adult life and had inculcated much of that identity, including that of being poor. Sheila's husband abused her and was in jail at the time of our interviews. Even though she was not Hispanic, the fact that she was married to a Hispanic man and was living among African Americans at the time colored her subjective experiences, much as it did those of Hispanic women. Among other topics, she told us about both her caseworker and the demographic realities of public housing as she saw them.

"My caseworker here at [the development], God I swear I hate her, she is deterring me....I put the transfer in [to move to a different housing development] but she says until your rent is paid, until this is done and this is done, we're not going to transfer you." Sheila told us how threatened she felt knowing that her husband knew where she lived and could find her when he is released from jail. She believed that if he found her he would return to hurt her or to try to take her children. In spite of these concerns, she said,

> They don't want you to leave here on a transfer. If you leave here, they want you to leave with the inability to reenter public housing. This is like the bottom, this is the ghetto of all ghettos, and they don't want you to move up. It's like, if you're here, you're bad. To me they want to keep you down.... In the Hispanic world, at least I speak their language, okay, and at least to them, I am not a total outcast. But to blacks in [this development] over there, I am taboo. Can you imagine me being the only person, my daughters being the only children in a completely ... I mean there are no Hispanics; ... [no] integration over there at all. I have no prejudices, but can you imagine us being the only white or only other race in those projects? Can you imagine what my daughters would go through? That's where she wanted to send me. They're worse there than they are here. Constant shooting, constant stabbings, drug wars ... so I am having a real hard time transferring.

This passage raises a troubling aspect of group identity and the inevitable conflict that results from competition for scarce resources. Competition among the poorest groups often led to intragroup tensions, and it was clear that some individuals, like Sheila, saw individuals from other groups or the neighborhoods in which they live as "worse" in some way. Other researchers have found similar patterns of group attribution among the poor. The cultural ecology of urban areas, in which the poorest neighborhoods are occupied by minority-group members, gives rise to intergroup tensions as members of different racial and ethnic groups vie for scarce local resources, such as housing, and limited public benefits (Wilson 1999).

In a period of increasing economic inequality, agendas based on race and ethnicity make effective intergroup coalition building difficult, but as we observed, group conflict only undermines the ability of those at the bottom to improve their lot (Wilson 1999). Yet it is a tragic reality of those who are forced to live in ethnically and racially segregated ghettos. Some writers have noted that material scarcity as well as political powerlessness have led to an increase in coalition politics as minority groups and the disenfranchised attempt to join forces (Browning, Marshall, and Tabb 2003). Such coalition building represents a hopeful and potentially positive response to minority-group powerlessness, but it is not always successful, and as we observed, the immediacy of one's frustration can easily be directed against the nearest people rather than the power elite.

Intergroup tensions emerged in all three cities. Just before and during the time of our study, rapid racial and ethnic changes were occurring in many neighborhoods, especially in San Antonio, and these were accompanied at various points by increased racial and ethnic tensions. In turn, these tensions, attitudes, and views of the racial and ethnic mapping in their communities affected what happened in welfare offices. One Hispanic respondent from Chicago reported that there was "a lot of racism against Hispanics. People who speak English [get] better treatment and shorter waiting times for appointments." Another respondent commented on the rudeness of the caseworkers that was directed against people who could not communicate well. She told us that she didn't know whether this reflected real discrimination or whether the caseworkers just got annoyed with anyone who couldn't speak English well. Reiterating a phrase we heard from several respondents in many contexts, she commented, "The staff act as though they were doing you the favor of giving you the medical card."

Another Hispanic respondent commented on the difference she perceived in the way black and Hispanic caseworkers treated clients depending on their race and ethnicity, and she explained why she preferred the Hispanics. She explained that one caseworker was a "prieta," clearly a derogatory term in this context that refers to dark skin color. She said that this caseworker was a "mean one, too." She preferred the "Latinos because they know what's up. . . . These people [the "prietos"], they treat you like nothing. . . . They've been pissing you off because of the way they act with you."

In Chicago, an African American mother commented, "They treat them [whites] like they may be down right now, but 'whities' will get back on their feet quicker." She explained that even the caseworker's voice and body language were different when they were dealing with people from different groups. "All the low-level workers are black, but their supervisors are white. The workers treat all of us bad, but the higher-ups look like they feel bad for the white families." Our white respondents also reflected on racial tensions in their communities. In Boston, one white mother told us about her impressions of the racial preferences she saw in Boston politics:

Well it [television] shows [the mayor] constantly opening a brand new ground or handing somebody keys to a new house that the neighbors got together and fixed up and everything. You see this all the time on that, that channel. And it's always Dorchester, Mattapan, and it's always a black family that's standing beside him. I've never once watched that program and seen a white person standing beside him.... Well, they know, because now they know that the black and the Hispanic community is the majority. They are not the minority, so definitely kiss their ass because you want their votes, you want them to be happy.

Respondents in San Antonio echoed many similar sentiments. Many felt that the race of their caseworker made a difference in how they were treated and that an applicant who was the same race as the caseworker was treated better or more fairly and got better results at the welfare office. In San Antonio, African American respondents often reported that in a city in which Hispanics were the majority, the city provided better services and supports to Hispanics than to blacks. In all three cities, both Hispanic and African American mothers assessed their caseworkers partly in terms of their race.

Again, although race and ethnicity were underlying themes of much of the discussion of housing, access to jobs, and treatment in the welfare office, it was poverty and the need to continually prove that one was poor and reaffirm one's status as a pauper in order to get desperately needed help that permeated our discussions with our respondents. Dealing with welfare agencies was often an exercise in futility, but more importantly it was a continuing confrontation with the reality of poverty and powerlessness. Like the mother we mentioned earlier, many of our mothers talked about the "ugliness" of their dealings with caseworkers and the humiliation that accompanied the application and recertification processes. Like all stereotypes of one group by another, the racist comments and caricatures we occasionally heard clearly reflected the frustrations that emerged as part of the conflict among powerless groups for limited benefits, including the caseworker's time. Poverty and powerlessness do not necessarily create allies among poor groups. As in other social strata, conflict over resources often brings out the worst in people.

Part of the powerlessness our respondents felt was expressed through a ghetto or barrio humor in which they poked fun at themselves and the system. One mother gave us examples of the kinds of jokes she makes about welfare stereotypes. She explained that people call the food stamp card "the Link," but she calls it the "Ghetto MasterCard – never leave home without it." She added, "Hey, when I was down at the office getting the whole package, the food stamps and everything, from month to month I was like, I'm a welfare queen."

Language and a lack of clarity in communication often represented a barrier to obtaining services and again underscored the power difference between agent and client, and this was a problem not just for those who were not fluent in English. One Hispanic mother in Boston explained that her welfare case had been closed when she did not understand exactly what the caseworker was asking for:

It happened to me on an occasion when certain information had been asked of me for Boston Housing, for the apartment. So the social worker did not make clear certain documents [that] she wanted. So I read the paper, and I sent her what [it] said to provide. Sometimes Hispanics [don't understand exactly], but it wasn't that I did not understand because I brought to her what I read. But she had a more specific document in mind than what I had sent her. So that's why then she sent me a notice where it said that they were going to close my case because I hadn't complied with providing all the documents that were asked of me. I went to the office [and] I had to fight for a hearing.

In the end, we came away with the realization that our respondents' poverty, in addition to denying them and their family needed basics for a decent life, also exposed them to humiliating reminders of their powerlessness and social marginality. As we have shown in the previous chapters, however, despite their relative powerlessness, few parents gave up and they did what was necessary, including enduring the humiliation of the application process and interactions with hostile bureaucrats, in order to ensure that their children received the best health care they could provide. When it came to their own health and health care, however, the system simply did not offer many options. The struggle for family health care coverage therefore was largely a struggle focused on children. As we will see in Chapter 7, a system based on employer-sponsored health insurance that provides publicly funded coverage only to the most impoverished adults places the health of many poor Americans at serious risk.

7

The Nonexistent Safety Net for Parents

For the parents in our study, one of the greatest threats to their children's health insurance coverage came as a result of their leaving the welfare rolls and going to work. As we have heard in the previous chapters, those parents who somehow managed to earn enough money to move the family above the poverty line ran the risk of losing Medicaid even for their younger children. The extension of Medicaid coverage to children in families with incomes well above the poverty line and the introduction of the State Children's Health Insurance Program (SCHIP) represent responses by Congress to a clearly irrational aspect of public health policy that penalized work and that left many working poor families without any source of health care coverage for their children. Unfortunately, even though Congress has partially addressed the problem that working poor families face in providing care to their children, it has done little to address the problem of the lack of coverage for their parents (Davidoff et al. 2004; Kaiser Commission on Medicaid and the Uninsured 2003).

Because of the lack of complete and comprehensive family coverage, many of the families in our study faced the harsh reality that some family members, very frequently the adults, had no health care coverage. As we have noted throughout, those families with incomes too high to qualify for Medicaid or SCHIP are at high risk of incomplete family coverage (Hanson 2001; Institute of Medicine 2002b). For parents, the lack of health coverage meant that they often did not get the medical care they needed, and they often experienced periods during which even serious problems went untreated. A study by the Henry J. Kaiser Family Foundation is only the most recent of a series of studies that show that women without health insurance coverage are less likely than those with coverage to seek medical care on a timely basis, to be referred to specialty care, or to receive important screening tests (Salganicoff, Ranji, and Wyn 2005). The Kaiser study, like our own, found the problem of restricted and incomplete access to be particularly serious among low-income and single women and Latinas. As we showed in Chapter 5, poor health and difficulties in getting preventive care and treatment for ongoing problems represent major roadblocks to employment that interfere with parents' ability to care for their families. There can be little doubt that for poor women, who are at the highest risk of poor health, the lack of health insurance is far more than a simple inconvenience. It has implications for the intergenerational transmission of poverty because it represents a major factor that keeps families trapped in low-income neighborhoods.

A Health Care Time Warp

During the twentieth century, mortality rates for all groups dropped and general health levels improved, largely as a result of the successful control of the chronic diseases of adulthood such as diabetes, hypertension, and obesity (Angel and Angel 2005; Freund, McGuire, and Podhurst 2003). Despite these overall improvements, however, serious disparities in health conditions and the risk of dying from those conditions remain (Kingston 2002; U.S. Department of Health and Human Services 2000). Improvements in the health of the poor lag behind those of the middle class by decades. Serious chronic diseases, such as diabetes, hypertension, and obesity, as well as other causes of impairment and death, continue to be more prevalent among low-income populations than among more affluent groups (Iannotta 2002; Institute of Medicine 2002a; Link and Phelan 1995). In addition, certain group-specific vulnerabilities are exacerbated by poverty to place members of those groups at a particularly elevated risk of serious debilitating illness. Mexican Americans, for example, suffer from extremely high levels of adult-onset diabetes, which, as the portrait that follows this introduction shows, is progressive and can result in serious life-threatening complications if not treated aggressively (Black, Ray, and

Markides 1999; Diehl and Stern 1989; Harris et al. 1998; Kuo et al. 2003; Stern et al. 1984; Wu et al. 2003).

Poverty is not only a threat to physical health but also undermines mental health. Individuals with chronic diseases such as diabetes, for example, frequently suffer from depression (Black, Markides, and Ray 1999). These simultaneous elevated physical and mental health risks among the poor underscore the fact that the mind and the body are intimately interconnected and also reveal the pervasive and pernicious influence of poverty and social disadvantage (Angel and Thoits 1987; Angel and Williams 2000). As we learned in Chapter 6, the increased physical and mental health risks are made even more serious by minority-group status and the discrimination that minority Americans must endure.

The appropriate management of diabetes, cardiovascular diseases, and other chronic conditions depends upon early diagnosis and diligent follow-up. Because the poor are less likely than middle-class Americans to have health insurance, they are more likely not to be diagnosed or to be diagnosed later in the disease process. Many chronic conditions, including diabetes and heart disease, have few early symptoms and are usually detected during routine examinations. The lack of health insurance reduces the probability of just such routine preventive care, increasing the probability that the disease will not be detected until it results in serious symptoms and functional limitations. Many individuals who suffer from such chronic conditions are often unaware of the source of their symptoms or their lack of general vitality.

Epidemiologists and health policy researchers are well aware of the fact that surveys that are based on self-reports of such chronic conditions can produce biased results. Individuals with serious conditions that have never been diagnosed because they do not receive routine care respond negatively to questions about whether a doctor has ever told them that they have the disease. Like many of our respondents, these individuals may experience symptoms such as headaches, dizziness, and a lack of energy, but because of a lack of health coverage they do not go to a doctor for treatment. As we have learned in earlier chapters, those individuals without coverage are very unlikely to have the personal resources to pay for even routine care out-of-pocket. Even if a poor person receives a diagnosis and a recommended treatment regimen, the high cost of complying with complicated dietary and medication regimens may prevent him or her from doing so. Individuals with few resources, especially if they have transportation difficulties, often fail to make the frequent follow-up visits that are necessary to control the disease.

The lack of a universal system of health care coverage therefore greatly increases health risks for the poor at the same time that it creates multiple barriers to access to adequate medical care. The lack of care undermines a parent's health and frequently contributes to an overall sense of a lack of control, diminished vitality, and the inability to perform important social roles. The fact that the poor have generally worse health than the middle class means that reference-group standards may also be affected. As we noted in Chapter 6, race and ethnicity assume a taken-for-granted quality that defines a group's social and economic experiences. Poor-group health levels can work in the same manner. The expectations for optimal levels of physical health and functioning that are typical of the middle class are unrealistic for poorer groups, potentially resulting in lower group expectations that feed into a complex interactive spiral of poor physical and mental health, inadequate health care, and lowered productivity (Angel and Thoits 1987). Let us begin with two case studies of mothers who had to forgo health care for fairly serious problems because they had no way to pay for it.

Teresa

Teresa, a divorced thirty-three-year-old Mexican American mother of three, lived in a subsidized apartment in a sprawling housing development on the west side of San Antonio. She had two daughters, ages eleven and twelve, and an infant son. We met the family through a caseworker who worked for a self-sufficiency program and who knew Teresa even though she was not enrolled in that particular program. We stayed in contact with the family for three years and conducted frequent interviews. Teresa's story illustrates the difficulties that adults, even those with serious medical problems, face in obtaining the care they need.

Teresa had suffered from adult-onset diabetes for ten years at the time she joined the study. Like Teresa, many Mexican Americans experience a very early onset of type II diabetes, which among the poor is associated with a poor diet, obesity, and a lack of exercise.

Unfortunately, the earlier the disease manifests itself, the longer it has to do its damage. Teresa's sister also had diabetes, and given the probable genetic predisposition among Mexican-origin individuals, the disease often affects several family members. The poverty in which Teresa lived undoubtedly contributed significantly to the onset of the disease and the course it took over the years. Diabetes is a chronic disease that requires constant vigilance in order to avoid extremely serious secondary problems, including heart disease, kidney failure, blindness, and peripheral nerve and blood vessel damage that can require the amputation of limbs. With proper management, which includes constant monitoring of one's blood sugar, close dietary control, and regular exercise, the ravages of the disease might be avoided. Without constant vigilance, they cannot.

The disease was the source of constant worry and many problems in Teresa's life. Despite the seriousness of her condition, however, she was unable to obtain all of the medical care she needed to deal with the disease and its consequences. Teresa's history of diabetes was long and complicated. It was often hard to tell whether she had ever received clear instructions concerning appropriate medication use or the appropriate diabetic diet from any of the physicians she had seen. She may, of course, simply have been noncompliant and not been following their advice. There was no way for us to know. As we got to know the family well, however, we realized that Teresa was not following the standard diabetic diet, which is low in sugars, salt, and fats. The family's meals, which Teresa shared, consisted of what many poor people eat, including prepared foods that are high in the components she should have been avoiding. We also suspected that she was not taking the correct dosage of her medication because she complained of numbness and dizziness. What we learned from our interactions with families in the study is that people on very limited budgets often take lower doses of prescription medications than they are prescribed in order to make the medicines last longer. Needless to say, such a practice seriously undermines the effectiveness of the treatment.

Despite the serious long-term consequences of poorly managed diabetes, Teresa was not able to get appointments to see a physician monthly as she had been advised, and her condition deteriorated during the course of the study. In our first interview in July 1999, Teresa reported that the doctor had recommended swimming as part of her treatment because there was a swimming pool at the development in which the family lived. Although she told us that she had been able to go to the pool a couple of times, taking care of her baby prevented her from swimming regularly.

At times Teresa seemed not to understand her medical condition or how it should be treated. Like many individuals with chronic diseases, she had tried many home remedies, but none had worked. Once she was diagnosed, which must have been well into the disease process, Teresa began taking pills to control her blood sugar. Within a year, the disease had worsened and she needed insulin injections. During a six-month follow-up interview in February 2002, she told us that she no longer took insulin because it made her feel worse. Instead, when she felt that her blood sugar was low, she would eat a piece of candy or drink a glass of orange juice. At our twelve-month follow-up interview with her, Teresa told us that she was again taking insulin.

At the time we recruited her into the study, Teresa was still receiving the Medicaid coverage for which she had qualified while she was pregnant with her infant son, and she was getting some financial assistance from the father of one of her daughters. She did not receive any assistance from her son's father and no longer had any contact with him because, as she told us without offering any specifics, he had molested one of the girls. After her last pregnancy, Teresa had experienced numbness in her legs, and by July had difficulty walking, but at the time she did not have a car. In order to get to her doctor's appointments or to appointments at the welfare office, she had to walk several blocks to the nearest bus stop.

Teresa's health problems were clearly compounded by those of her children. Despite the obvious urgency of her own medical problems, like so many other parents she focused her time and resources on getting them care first. In addition to forcing Teresa to ignore or postpone her own care, getting care for her children placed real physical demands on her body that exacerbated her condition and drained her energy. Even with her strong desire to do right by everyone in the family, there was only so much she could do. Because of the difficulties she had with transportation and the difficulty she had walking, she had a hard time keeping medical appointments with her own or her children's regular doctor. Instead, she would often take the children to one of the local clinics to which she could more easily travel by bus.

A year after our first interview, and as her condition deteriorated, Teresa developed glaucoma and black spots appeared in her visual field. Despite her vision problems and the clear financial sacrifice, she bought a car in order to get to and from the jobs that she could find. Her legs continued to bother her, and her fingers, hands, and feet began to ache. By this point she was taking three different oral medications in addition to insulin, although we were never certain what those were. She also had been told that her diabetes had affected her organs, but she offered no details. Soon after that she reported that her kidneys were severely damaged. As her health continued to deteriorate, her medical care and medication use remained episodic.

The family's life was clearly consumed by health problems and the need to find care, and Teresa often had a hard time understanding or complying with treatment recommendations. Both of her daughters had been diagnosed with learning disabilities and had been placed in special education classes. The younger daughter also had attention deficit hyperactivity disorder (ADHD) and had been prescribed Ritalin. As with her own diabetes, Teresa seemed uncertain as to how to deal with her daughter's problems. The Ritalin prescription called for the drug to be administered three times a day, but according to Teresa it caused the girl to lose her appetite and become sluggish. In order to reduce those side effects, Teresa decided to have the girl take the Ritalin only while at school so that she would not "throw fits" and disrupt the class. She seemed either unaware of the need to comply with the specific prescription requirements or chose not to do so for reasons that were not really clear. While we were in contact with them, the family's problems only got worse. By May 2000, the boy was showing signs of developmental delay; he could crawl but not stand by himself. In addition, he had developed asthma.

Teresa had a tenth-grade education and had been struggling to complete her GED before her son was born. Unfortunately, her poor health interfered with her education as well as her ability to find work, and she was unable to finish the course. Despite not having a degree, she found employment as a nursing assistant and was able to leave welfare for a while. As was the case for many other mothers, however, the job was only temporary, and Teresa stopped working during her pregnancy because she was increasingly ill with her diabetes and bronchitis. Although the nursing assistant position paid slightly above minimum wage and was full-time, it provided no benefits for her or her children, and while she was pregnant she became eligible for and received Medicaid and TANF.

For adults with serious disabilities, Social Security insurance provides more reliable health care coverage and qualifies a family for TANF. Teresa began the process of applying for Social Security insurance support for herself in mid-1999. After her younger daughter's hyperactivity was diagnosed, she also applied for supplemental security income (SSI) for the girl. These applications were not immediately successful and, as is the case with most SSI applications, Teresa had to make several administrative appearances and spend a great deal of time and effort finding and presenting documentation before the two cases were approved. Meanwhile, because of the TANF work requirements, Teresa was continually reminded that she was required to look for work for several hours per week, a requirement that she could not always meet because of her own health problems, her children's health problems, and the administrative struggles required to deal with them. In 1999, while she was pregnant, she was threatened with being sanctioned for not working, but she successfully fought penalties by proving that she was five months pregnant. She knew that although she would have a grace period after the birth, she would again be required to look for work.

Meanwhile, in early December 1999, well before the disability cases were settled, Teresa and her children moved into a shelter for awhile because she did not have money for rent. During this period when the family was homeless, her welfare benefits were cut even further because her oldest child missed a week of school. Through it all, Teresa continued to try to get medical care for her illness and to qualify for government support, but out of desperation she began to look for work even though she anticipated that once she was employed she would lose all assistance, including her medical coverage.

Because she had received training as a nurse assistant, Teresa felt certain that she could find employment, but she had serious anxieties about the job's physical demands, which included lifting patients, and initially she sought other work. She found a job cleaning up after games at the local sports arena, but she quit that job after only three weeks. That job paid only $5.50 an hour and required that she work at night. Teresa could not find anyone to take care of her children while she worked the evening shift. In addition, the job was physically challenging, especially given her health problems. The job finally ended with her son's sudden illness and hospitalization with pneumonia. Even after her son recovered, Teresa decided not to return to the night job.

By February 2000, Teresa's daughter had qualified for SSI and she became eligible for a number of new programs and medications. Meanwhile, Teresa's application for Social Security insurance continued to be denied. In December 2000, she told us that her vision was deteriorating because of her glaucoma and cataracts. However, despite her deteriorating health, her physician would not certify her disability status because, according to her, he viewed her problems as arising from weight gain and he thought that she should be able to control the symptoms by losing weight. By now Teresa had a car so, although driving with impaired sight was a risk, she drove to her monthly checkups. Her new job as a nursing assistant, however, created a different problem. Because the job did not provide sick leave, she missed many of the appointments even though she had transportation because she could not afford to take time off from work.

By February 2002, Teresa had to quit working again. She was having trouble standing or walking because her legs would become numb and collapse under her. She told us that a pinched nerve in her back had caused the problem. Because of the pain, she remained seated much of the day and used a cane to walk. The nursing care company could not keep her on under these circumstances, and the family again became dependent on welfare.

Finally, following the numerous hearings that are typical of Social Security insurance applications, Teresa was approved in August 2002. She told us that she believed that she had been approved only because she had been sent to specialists recommended by the caseworkers. As a result of receiving these funds, Teresa made immediate changes in the treatment of her diabetes. She told us at our twelve-month follow-up interview that she had begun to receive treatment at a new clinic in her neighborhood and even attended "diabetes classes" to learn about proper diet and exercise for diabetics. The clinic also offered exercise classes, but because the location at which they were offered was too far away, Teresa exercised by walking around the neighborhood instead.

By fall 2002, Teresa was trying to find out how she could make her house wheelchair-accessible because she believed that having a wheelchair would make her house chores and taking care of her youngest child easier. Although she continued to drive, she was increasingly dependent on her eldest daughter, who had a learner's permit. At the time of our last contact with Teresa and her family, they were clearly better off than when we met them, largely because of the Social Security insurance and supplemental security income that Teresa and her daughter were receiving. Nonetheless, it was clear that their struggles to maintain health care coverage for other members of the family would continue and that Teresa's health problems would continue to undermine her efforts to get ahead. Although she was a relatively young woman, Teresa's body had been ravaged by her diabetes and its complications. Like so many other parents, she had neglected her own health in her struggle to get care for her children and maintain a home for them. Teresa's case clearly illustrates the fact that poor families face greater threats to their health and are more likely to suffer from the long-term consequences of illness that might be avoided by early and adequate medical care. Without coverage, that care is often unavailable, and poor health undermines its victims' educational ambitions, their attempts to stay employed, and their effectiveness as parents.

Yvonne's Health Problems

Yvonne, the Mexican American mother of five whom we met in the last chapter, offered another poignant example of a low-income adult's dilemma when it comes to her own health care. In the last chapter, we recounted the many problems that Yvonne faced and showed how her poverty and her minority-group identity contributed to the difficulties she had in dealing with them, which in turn increased her depression and demoralization. As was so often clear in our study, the health risks associated with poverty manifest themselves both physically and emotionally, and as with Yvonne we encountered much depression and more serious mental illness. Yvonne's demoralization was fueled in large part by poor health and the difficulties in getting care for herself and everyone else in the family. She suffered from the long-term effects of a childhood spinal injury for which she took medication in order to control the pain. Getting the medication on a regular basis was a problem because of her lack of insurance. Adults like Yvonne, who do not qualify for Social Security insurance, must rely on Medicaid when they can get it and charity when they cannot. A few nongovernmental organizations (NGOs) offer assistance with psychiatric medications, but their capacity is limited given the magnitude of the need.

Yvonne also suffered frequent bouts of acute illness that may well have been both the cause and the result of her generally low vitality but was no doubt exacerbated by a lifetime in poverty. As we recounted in the last chapter, she suffered from a strong allergic reaction to flea bites, an easily avoidable side effect of her unsatisfactory and unsanitary living conditions. She not only could not move to better housing but also had difficulty getting the medication to treat the problem. Yvonne's mother had been diagnosed with AIDS, one of the few conditions that qualify one for Social Security insurance because of its chronic and devastating nature. Her mother's AIDS was added evidence of the pervasive health risks faced by individuals in Yvonne's social class, and her mother's illness clearly added to Yvonne's sense of hopelessness. To deal with her ongoing depression, Yvonne needed therapy and medication that she again was not always able to get.

Teresa and Yvonne's cases illustrate the severity of the health problems that parents in low-income families experience and the difficulty they face in getting care for themselves. Our interviews made it clear that poor adults are seriously neglected by our current public and private systems of health care financing. It was also clear that this situation creates and perpetuates serious health problems that can undermine an adult's productivity and parenting capacities. Pregnant and nursing mothers are covered by Medicaid, as are working-age adults with severely disabling conditions. Few others except for the truly destitute qualify for any public program, however, and when they become ill they are forced to rely on emergency rooms, public clinics, and nongovernmental charitable organizations for whatever treatment they can get. As Teresa's case showed, however, such charitable organizations are rarely equipped to deal with complex or chronic health problems.

Health problems pervaded our interviews with respondents. Even when the topic of our interviews was not health, health problems and their consequences came up frequently in discussions of other areas of family life. Health truly is wealth, and our families had little of either. The mechanisms by which poverty undermines a parent's health, as well as their parenting capacities and their productive potential, are hardly mysterious. By now the pervasive disparities in health among racial and ethnic groups, as well as their causes, are fairly well understood (U.S.

Department of Health and Human Services 2000). Most are related to the serious inequalities that characterize our society and our health care system. Again our study makes obvious the serious contradictions and inequalities in our current health care and welfare policies. The fact that individuals who play by the rules and do their best to become self-sufficient are placed at elevated risk of poor health and inadequate health care is a national tragedy.

The Complex Health Care System for the Poor

As our case studies have shown, the health care system for the poor provides anything but seamless care. Low-income families must negotiate a complex and confusing system that includes multiple sources of care and different providers. It includes emergency rooms, clinics, charitable care, and private physicians. As a consequence, the system does not provide continuity of care, one of the hallmarks of high-quality health care. Poor families are not assigned to, nor are they permitted to choose, a single clinic or health care provider who might coordinate all of their preventive and acute care. Rather than simply going to a usual care provider, poor families first have to meet eligibility criteria and then find a provider who will accept their coverage. Often, those providers did not practice nearby, and, as we have shown, getting to a provider with whom one can make an appointment and who will accept Medicaid can consume a great deal of time.

Many of our families had trouble finding a doctor who would accept Medicaid as the sole payment for services because reimbursements are so low. Even once they found a doctor willing to accept Medicaid patients, however, many parents had difficulties juggling their work schedules in order to keep an appointment for themselves or a child, especially when several visits were required. When they finally got to the doctor, their problems did not end because after receiving a diagnosis and treatment plan, they often found that they did not have the money to pay for over-the-counter or nonpharmaceutical items that were not covered by Medicaid. Hopefully, the growing use of HMOs by state Medicaid programs will address some of the problems of continuity of care.

As a consequence of the current fragmented and incomplete system of coverage, families faced frequent periods when one or another member of the household was without coverage and when not everyone's health care needs could be addressed. This lack of consistent health insurance forced families to triage and make difficult decisions about which family member's health care needs came first, especially if the family had to pay out-of-pocket or if only the youngest children were covered by Medicaid. In these cases, the needs of other family members, especially those of the parents, simply had to wait. These coverage shortcomings were not just personal and isolated problems that some of our study families encountered. They were very common and arose from fundamental shortcomings in our health care financing system that almost inevitably result in incomplete and episodic health care coverage and compromised access to care for various family members. The insecurity that results from an endless scramble to maintain as much coverage as possible and to get access to medical services seriously affected many other aspects of family routines and stability.

Our interviews revealed the rapidity and frequency with which family members cycled ("churned") among various public programs in a process that almost invariably left parents uncovered. Although the poor receive charitable care even at for-profit hospitals, their tie to the health care system is tenuous and lacks the certainty and continuity that middle-class Americans enjoy. Although they receive care for the most pressing problems, that care often comes late in the disease process. As we have noted, the poor and minorities face an elevated risk of death from cancer, heart disease, and the other leading causes of death (Institute of Medicine 2004), due in part to their susceptibility to diseases and in part to their tendency to receive health care relatively late. The care they receive is less regular and dependable and is often inferior to that received by adequately insured middle-class Americans (Institute of Medicine 2001; Institute of Medicine 2002a; Institute of Medicine 2002b). What we witnessed was an ongoing struggle for adequate and complete health care in which families face a kaleidoscope of different possibilities that shift frequently and rarely meet all of a family's needs.

Evidence from the Survey: Incomplete Family Coverage

The extent of the lack of coverage that we witnessed in the ethnography led us to wonder about the factors at the family and individual

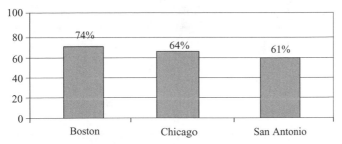

FIGURE 7.1. Percentage of households in which the caregiver and all children in the household are covered by city

levels that might be associated with the lack of full family coverage. It is clear that the basic problem is structural and results from the fact that our employment-based health care insurance system leaves out large numbers of families and family members. As we have seen, however, those families do not represent a random cross section of the entire population. They are disproportionately minority. In order to answer the question about what other characteristics of our families increased or decreased the probability that they would have full family coverage, we turn to the survey. Again we must remember that the survey represents a snapshot, and the ethnography made it clear that much more instability than is apparent from the survey lies below the surface. The fact that many families cycle on and off Medicaid means that the total period during which someone in the family lacks coverage during the course of a year is probably higher than one might recognize on the basis of survey data. A question in the first wave of the survey concerning whether there had been a period during the last year when either the caregiver or the focal child was without health coverage includes much missing data. The question is probably too difficult to answer simply given the volatility in coverage that the ethnography revealed.

In the second wave of the survey, we asked about the health insurance status of every member of the household. This information makes it possible for us to investigate the extent and correlates of the lack of complete family coverage. In what follows, we compare those households in which all members have some form of health care coverage and those in which someone has no coverage. Figure 7.1 presents the overall patterns by city and reflects the impact of state policy differences

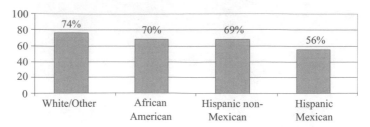

FIGURE 7.2. Percentage of households in which the caregiver and all children in the household are covered by caregiver's race or Hispanic ethnicity

on household coverage. In Boston, everyone was covered in 74 percent of families, but in Chicago only 64 percent and in San Antonio only 61 percent of families had full coverage. This means that nearly 40 percent of households in San Antonio included someone with no health care coverage of any sort at the time of the survey. Even in Boston, with its more generous system for poor families, over 32 percent of households included someone with no coverage.

Once again, these point estimates refer to the date of the survey and, given the volatility of coverage, they probably underestimate the number of families that at some time during a year include someone with no coverage. As we noted in Chapter 5, part of the explanation for lower rates of incomplete family coverage in Boston probably lies in the fact that more parents were employed in that city than in Chicago or San Antonio, but even in Boston employment often reduces the probability of public coverage for children as well as adults.

The survey provided some further insights into the characteristics of households without full coverage. For example, Figure 7.2 reveals the serious vulnerability associated with Mexican origin that we discussed earlier. Although African American and Hispanic, non-Mexican families, a category that includes Puerto Ricans, Dominicans, and others, were less likely to have full family coverage than non-Hispanic white families, Mexican-origin families were far less likely than any other group to be fully covered. Nearly half of all Mexican-origin families included someone who was not covered. The reason is unclear, although many potential explanations have been offered, including the large number of undocumented aliens in this population, larger family size, discrimination, difficulties with English, and other cultural barriers. The ethnography showed that dealing with the Medicaid

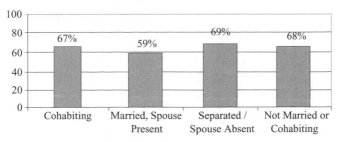

FIGURE 7.3. Percentage of households in which the caregiver and all children are covered by caregiver's marital status

bureaucracy is difficult and is made more so by language and other cultural barriers. Such explanations are made more plausible by the fact that citizenship status appears to be an important variable as well. Among Mexican-origin individuals, citizenship issues are highly salient and sensitive, and it is clear that some community members, both legal and illegal, believe that using welfare of any sort might have negative repercussions either for some family member's ability to become a citizen or simply by attracting the attention of the authorities.

Other important correlates of full family coverage emerged from the survey, and the ethnographic data that follow provide deeper insight into these factors. Figure 7.3 shows that two-parent households (that is, those in which the male spouse is present) were less likely to have full family coverage than households headed by women in which no male was present. This reflects the marriage penalty associated with Medicaid. As the ethnography revealed, the presence of a male in the household can be a very mixed blessing. If he contributes to household income and stability, and especially if he provides health insurance, his presence is a clear advantage. If, as we so often found, his contribution is sporadic or relatively small but his presence results in the loss of benefits, including Medicaid, his impact on household well-being may well be mixed or negative. In such cases, the possibility of a stable relationship is undermined. Clearly, many nonmarital cohabiting relationships are unstable, as our survey data showed, but the marriage penalty that is part of our current welfare policy does not help. Men who cannot provide income or health care to their families are denied a source of satisfaction and are forced into a situation of having to leave or penalizing those they might like to help. The help that men

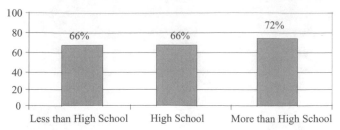

FIGURE 7.4. Percentage of households in which the caregiver and all children are covered by caregiver's education

provide is often in-kind or hidden, as we discussed in Chapter 6. Such arrangements are demeaning and further undermine the man's basic sense of worth.

The major objective of welfare reform, of course, was to get families off the TANF rolls as quickly as possible, preferably by increasing their earnings capacity so that they leave permanently and become self-sufficient. Such an objective clearly requires an increase in productivity and access to better jobs, which results, in turn, from more education and better training, human capital inputs that are expensive and time consuming. A central focus of most antipoverty programs has historically been on general education and specific employment-related skills. Parents with higher levels of education possess human capital that translates directly into higher incomes and an increased probability that all family members, including themselves, will have health coverage (Carrasquillo, Carrasquillo, and Shea 2000; Heck and Parker 2002; Perloff 1999).

Even in our relatively poorly educated sample, as the caregivers' education increased, the probability that all members of the household had health coverage increased as well. Figure 7.4 shows that in families in which the parent has some post–high school education or training, the probability of full family coverage increases. Clearly, increased education and job training would help raise many families out of poverty, increasing their access to health insurance and high-quality health care. Part of the rhetoric of welfare reform and welfare policy historically has focused on education and training. Although some states have provided interesting alternatives for training and education, most such efforts are relatively short-term, and the work-first philosophy of current policy focuses on getting parents to apply for jobs and to take whatever employment they can find even when it offers no long-term possibilities for the development of job skills.

These descriptive findings from the survey highlight some of the major factors that influence health insurance coverage. State policy, marital status, and race and ethnicity emerged as important predictors of health insurance coverage that were not accounted for by other factors. In multivariate analyses of the predictors of coverage for the focal child and for the family as a whole that have been published elsewhere, these characteristics remain significant even when other factors are introduced (Angel, Frias, and Hill 2005). In those analyses, Mexican-origin families are less likely to have full family coverage than any other group. They also show that families of noncitizens are less likely to have full coverage than families of parents who were born in the United States and that households in which the father is present have lower levels of family coverage, again revealing a clear marriage penalty in Medicaid.

Constrained Rationality

As is the case for middle-class families, the choices that our low-income parents made were rational and intended to optimize their own and their children's welfare. Those choices, however, are seriously constrained by their lack of resources and the administrative and practical problems that are structured into highly bureaucratized, means-tested government programs. For parents in our study, choices about their own health care coverage and medical care use were constrained by the fact that they had almost no options. Unlike the middle class, the decisions concerning family health care coverage that the working poor make are not confined to the start of a new job, when one is offered a choice as part of one's benefit package. Rather than making a choice concerning family coverage at the beginning of a job and updating it on an annual basis or when one's family status changes, the unemployed and the working poor engage in never-ending attempts to get and keep basic coverage and to maintain contact with the health care system, sometimes on an illness-to-illness basis.

For the most part, the problems with health care coverage for both adults and children that we identified in the study resulted from the episodic nature of service-sector employment and the fact that the jobs for which our respondents qualified rarely offered affordable benefits either for the employee or his or her dependents. Families also experienced serious barriers inherent in the application and recertification process for Medicaid and other public programs and the fact that such programs only cover adults in special circumstances. Our ethnographic interviews offer unique insights into how these problems cumulate to undermine access to stable family health care. Ongoing surveys, such as the Current Population Survey (CPS) conducted by the U.S. Census Bureau, clearly document the extent of the problem of the lack of health insurance coverage in the United States. In 2003, for example, forty-five million individuals had no health insurance (DeNavas-Walt, Proctor, and Mills 2004). What surveys and one-time cross-sectional interview studies do not reveal, however, is the extent of the problem of incomplete and episodic coverage and the difficulty it causes in other areas of family life, including employment. Incomplete and inconsistent family coverage affects families in ways that our ethnographic interviews allow us to begin to understand. What our interviews demonstrate is that the instability of health care coverage is an integral part of the more pervasive instability in the lives of poor and near-poor families that separates them from the middle class and undermines their earnest efforts to get ahead.

In all three cities, mothers reported health conditions that went untreated or treatments that consisted of home remedies or other alternative care. Recall that Teresa attempted to deal with her diabetes using various home remedies. The use of home remedies and alternative therapies is quite common, and many middle-class diabetics with adequate health care coverage also try alternative treatments, but it was clear that for Teresa the cost and the difficulty in complying with the standard medically prescribed regimen was her major motivation. In addition to forcing them to use often ineffective home remedies, the inability to see a doctor or to pay for expensive prescription drugs led many adults in our study to reuse old medications or to borrow medications prescribed for someone else. One Chicago mother reported that she was treating herself for a dental infection using antibiotics that she had received for some other purpose. She had no dental coverage and could not afford to seek treatment from a dentist.

The problem is particularly serious in the case of chronic conditions that require ongoing medication. Chronic conditions such as diabetes, hypertension, and heart disease can only be managed, not cured. One must take medications and comply with a treatment program for the rest of one's life. Mental health problems are similar in that they require long-term supportive drug therapy. For such conditions, even when adults in the study managed to initially obtain their prescriptions, they could never be sure that they would be able to pay for refills. In San Antonio, one of the mothers, who suffered from a debilitating depression, worried constantly that she would not be able to afford the antidepressant medication that allowed her to work and carry out her parenting responsibilities. Without the medication, she could hardly function. Although we heard of private charitable sources that help with such medications, we did not actually come into contact with them. Even in Boston, where most of our sample had some form of health care coverage, mothers still reported lapses in their coverage because of bureaucratic mishaps as well as a lack of access to certain types of care, including dental and eye care.

Elizabeth

The case of Elizabeth, a young non-Hispanic white mother of two daughters, and one of the few non-Hispanics in our ethnographic sample, reveals the ways in which policy-driven barriers contribute to the incomplete nature of the health care that parents can acquire. It also illustrates the fact that the problems our respondents encountered were largely a function of their lack of resources and powerlessness in relation to the health care system rather than simply a reflection of race or Hispanic ethnicity. Elizabeth's daughters were three and four years old, and after leaving Texas to live in Florida for several weeks she had spent a great deal of time and effort recertifying for TANF when she returned to Texas. Elizabeth had accumulated a great deal of debt for past medical bills and had no idea of how she would ever pay it off. She owed between three and four hundred dollars for services for her daughters, and she was not even sure how much she owed for her own medical expenses. She simply tried not to think about it because there was nothing she could do. She told us that she used to receive bills in the mail but they had stopped coming, probably because she had moved to Florida.

Before the family's TANF and the children's Medicaid were reinstated after she returned from Florida, Elizabeth experienced a serious health crisis related to gastroenteritis. As we found time and time again, for Elizabeth, as for most families with no economic reserves and no health insurance, illnesses that might have been routine with adequate coverage precipitated a crisis. Because she could not ignore the problem, Elizabeth had been forced to pay over $200 for her initial diagnosis and prescriptions and, as a consequence, had not been able to pay her rent for the month of August. Because the problem did not clear up, Elizabeth had to be hospitalized and then had to stay home for several weeks. During this entire period she had no health care coverage. Despite considerable pain and suffering, Elizabeth was determined not to go deeper into debt and was especially determined not to risk her children's housing arrangement by again spending rent money on her own medical care. Driven by desperation and by her parental responsibilities, she delayed her hospitalization until she had completed her own Medicaid recertification.

Once Elizabeth had successfully completed the recertification process and after she received her medical treatment, she faced yet another problem. Although Medicaid paid for her hospital stay, once she was discharged Medicaid only paid for three prescription drugs per month. Elizabeth understood that after the first month she would be able to receive unlimited prescriptions, but she found the restrictions both mystifying and upsetting because she needed the prescriptions most when she was ill and not after she recovered. Again, we can only relay what Elizabeth told us and cannot be sure whether she was correct in her understanding of the situation. Clearly, her lack of clear understanding itself reflected some real confusion in a system that we as researchers often found bewildering and irrational.

Later in the study, Elizabeth again lost her Medicaid. This fact came out in one of our interviews with her when she commented on how useful the grocery store gift certificates we gave her had been because she could use them to help pay for the prescriptions she needed in order to manage the depression she had experienced off and on over the previous ten years. With Elizabeth, as with other women in the study, occasionally the depth of the demoralization they experienced emerged unexpectedly or indirectly as in this reflection on her depression that appeared to have become a matter-of-fact reality of her life. Elizabeth dealt with her depression as best she could, and because she could never put together the money for a full month's prescription, she told us that she brought in ten or twenty dollars each time she could get the money together to buy a few more days of her medical treatment.

Of course, as we have noted and as some critics of expanded programs for the poor point out, charitable or low-cost care is available to poor adults from nongovernmental organizations, and many sick adults seek care in emergency departments once they experience a crisis. In all three cities, including San Antonio, there were some clinics that took poor patients, even without Medicaid. However, as we have noted before, the ability of these clinics to deal with chronic or serious conditions is limited. They do not have the resources to deal with patients with conditions such as the diabetes and severe asthma that are so prevalent in the neighborhoods in which our respondents lived. One mother in San Antonio, who had recently been diagnosed with diabetes, explained how her increasing illness led to difficulties in finding care. The interviewer asked her where she was accustomed to getting medical care, and she replied,

Yes, it's a clinic. As a matter of fact, it's free; you don't have to worry about Medicaid. It just takes people who may be poor, who can't afford [to pay for health care]. I went there because it was convenient. It was so close to the house. But, they couldn't even see me any more. They said, "Oh, no. You're going to need more health care because you have diabetes."

The real tragedy that any close examination of the health care needs of poor adults reveals is, as we have shown, the fact that often aspects of their working conditions, their family and network responsibilities, their living conditions, and other environmental factors create inescapable health risks that lead to illnesses that frequently go years without treatment. As we have also documented, and as other studies have confirmed, late diagnosis and incomplete or inadequate treatment result in poorer health outcomes (Institute of Medicine 2001; Institute of Medicine 2002a). One mother described how the mental health problems she suffered as the result of what she claimed was a work-related illness went untreated for three years while she struggled to find a way to qualify for the necessary services. Early in the illness, she had received some workmen's compensation, but that had stopped. As she explained,

I was a telephone operator, and our air-conditioning vents were hooked up to three other places: one that made glue, one that cleaned airplane parts, and one that made another chemical. We were breathing that and didn't know that we were breathing it. So for a long period of time I couldn't read. I taught myself to read, to write, and to understand again. I want to go back to school because some of the things I don't remember. I could speak Spanish fluently and I don't remember how. And sign language, I don't [know]. So I want to take those courses again.... All these many years that I worked for the system, and I worked and had never been on assistance. There was no help for me until I finally got my disability, which took....I got hurt in ninety-four, and I got disability in ninety-seven. There was no help whatsoever in between. I've always...worked.

Some Final Thoughts: A Parent's Dilemma

Our study corroborated a large body of previous research that identifies several family and parental risk factors for poverty and incomplete family health care coverage. Low education, poor health, inescapable family responsibilities, service-sector employment, part-time work, and more increase the likelihood of poverty and reduce the likelihood of complete family coverage. These characteristics basically define the heavily black and Latino populations of low-resource urban neighborhoods. Of course, although it is possible to identify individual and family characteristics that are associated with incomplete health coverage, the association reflects more than individual choices and behaviors. The fact that the poor consist disproportionately of families of color provides strong evidence that opportunities for material and social success are structurally determined in ways that penalize blacks and Latinos.

A major tragedy that we observed was that the structural vulnerabilities that reduce a parent's physical and emotional resources are the same vulnerabilities that undermine their ability to be the high-quality role models for their children that they would like to be. Optimal parenting requires time, material resources, and self-esteem. The circumstances in which our families survive undermined all of those. As we have seen in previous chapters, family structure, a parent's level of education, their employment status, and the stability of the job they hold, as well as other aspects of family life that are related to family stability, are also related to the physical and mental functioning of its members. For the poor, their lack of resources means that moves between cities or states, or even between neighborhoods, that are often necessary because of unavoidable housing, work, and welfare changes directly affect the emotional climate of the family and a parent's effectiveness.

Our study also corroborated national statistics that show that employment alone is not enough to ensure full family coverage. Most uninsured children live in households with one or more employed adults (Perloff 1999). Employment often does not even provide health care coverage to the worker. At the lowest rungs on the occupational hierarchy, employment often leaves a family worse off than it might be if the parents were unemployed. Our data also revealed that the marriage penalty that is still part of Medicaid and other public programs further penalizes intact families and couples that attempt to stay together. Despite a fairly universal desire to support marriage and two-parent families, current Medicaid policy imposes a serious marriage penalty on poor two-parent households (Rolett et al. 2001).

Of course, some members of the families we studied engaged in behaviors that were detrimental to their long-term health and welfare and that undermined their chances for social or economic mobility. Drug abuse, criminal acts, and irresponsible sexual behavior are the frequent focus of critics of welfare who blame it for the rise in nonmarital pregnancy and the extensive social disorganization of our inner cities. There can be little doubt that the poor can behave as self-destructively and irresponsibly as members of the middle class. Our objective is not to excuse irresponsible behavior but to point out how social structures and irrational bureaucratic rules increase the likelihood of such behavior. Individuals with little hope for the future often find solace in immediate pleasures. It was clear that other aspects of the situations in which our families lived besides welfare worked against family stability.

Stable long-term relationships between parents were almost nonexistent in our study, and many women had children from different men. Few of these men provided health insurance even for their own children. Although the men's relationship with their families was often casual and unpredictable, many fathers did provide some income or help of some other sort to their children. In many ways, they did as much as they realistically could; it just was not enough. The ever-present and irrational reality of the situation in which our families found themselves was that if a male contributed too much and if that fact became obvious to the welfare agency, and especially if he was living in the household, the family lost essential services. Although it is clearly reasonable to expect men to support their families, the all-or-nothing approach that characterizes current policy struck us as counterproductive. As for the women in our study, small increments toward self-sufficiency often resulted in large losses because of inflexible and irrational rules. In this context, the expectation that a father could provide such a high-priced good as health care coverage is simply unrealistic.

Other irrationalities in the system that have been well documented also undermined our families' attempts to get ahead. Welfare has always been criticized for what was a nearly 100 percent implicit tax rate, which refers to the situation in which a person loses a dollar of support for every dollar earned. Such a tax is clearly a disincentive to leave welfare and a serious penalty for working. If a family also loses health care coverage, the system clearly discourages employment and marriage. Because of the clearly illogical nature of these disincentives, many states have changed the rules so that a dollar earned does not result in a dollar of benefits lost. In the case of marriage, however, the illogical and counterproductive nature of the rules remains. Unless a father can carry a large proportion of the burden of support for the family, his presence probably does more harm than good. Few of the fathers in our study could live up to this responsibility, and they and their families were penalized for partial efforts.

Part of the complexity of minority-group status and identity that we dealt with in Chapter 6 relates to the interaction of these separate vulnerabilities, which together create major barriers that poor families must overcome if they are to advance economically. With so many forces working against their ability to earn enough to survive on and to save, the task is daunting. In addition, these forces all work against the probability that a family could obtain health care coverage through work. African American and Hispanic parents face elevated risks to their own and their children's health and to their overall well-being, not because of the fact that they are minority-group members per se but because their minority status places them in a disadvantaged position in multiple domains relative to majority-group Americans. Hispanic ethnicity also reduces the likelihood of health coverage because of the fact that marriage rates and the proportion of two-parent households are higher among these groups, which subjects them to the marriage penalty.

African Americans and Hispanics have lower levels of education on average than non-Hispanic whites and are therefore more likely to be employed in low-wage jobs with no benefits. Clearly, improving their employability and their access to health care coverage requires education and training programs, which in reality receive only lip service in current welfare policy. Other access barriers to health care that are as yet poorly understood remain. As we have documented throughout, although Hispanics are more likely than non-Hispanic whites to qualify for public programs because of low income, as a group they continue to be seriously underinsured (Angel et al. 2001; Berk, Albers, and Schur 1996; Elixhauser et al. 2002; Flores et al. 1998; Flores et al. 2002; Hubble et al. 1991; Thamer and Richard 1997). The situation is particularly serious for immigrants and those who are not fluent in English (Carrasquillo, Carrasquillo, and Shea 2000; Granados et al. 2001; Ku and Waidmann 2003).

Given the growing instability in family health insurance that accompanies reductions in employer-sponsored plans and growing budgetary crises in public coverage, in the future a larger proportion of even working- and middle-class parents and children will experience periods without health insurance. As our study reveals, even children with health insurance at any particular moment are likely to experience periods during which they have no insurance. As the extent of coverage offered even to the insured decreases and as states find themselves facing ever more burdensome Medicaid budgets, more and more families will find that they have incomplete coverage. For the families in our study, the health care that both children and adults received was determined by the coverage offered under Medicaid. For the most part, this coverage did not include full dental or eye care. In San Antonio, as we saw, it also meant doing without some of the prescription medicine one might need.

Instability and Its Consequences

We end this chapter by returning to a core theme of the entire project. The lack of opportunities generally, and the lack of health insurance in particular, make it very difficult for families that cycle in and out of employment and on and off public programs to get ahead. The fact that many middle-class Americans began with nothing and worked their way up the economic ladder makes some observers unsympathetic to the plight of the families we studied. America, after all, is a nation of opportunities, and the common wisdom is that with diligence and hard work almost anyone, regardless of race or ethnicity, should be able to achieve at least a decent standard of living on their own. On the other hand, individuals who abuse drugs, who fail to take advantage of educational opportunities, or who are sexually careless should expect to fail. Women who have several children from different men and who have not completed high school can appear to be, and often are, irresponsible and careless.

Yet the poor are with us and some, including those with major drug habits, may be unsalvageable. There is little disagreement that individuals should be held responsible for their own actions and behaviors. Fathers who do not support their children deserve little respect or sympathy. Yet what administrative data and even our survey do not fully reveal but becomes more obvious from ethnographic data is the impact of the *instability* in the lives of these families and the ways in which it traps them in poverty. A large part of that instability, especially for minority families, is not of their making. Nor can numerical data show the hopelessness that accompanies dependency and the penalties that one suffers for sincere efforts to get ahead. In the public media, poverty has always been portrayed as a personal failure, and the poor have historically been stigmatized.

Today, nobody goes to the poorhouse, and the basic safety net of services has become a permanent part of the modern welfare state. Yet this safety net has characteristics that led even many liberals to accept welfare reform. Earnest and realistic attempts to act responsibly and improve oneself are undermined by the system itself. Whereas irresponsibility should clearly be punished, good behavior should not. Most of the parents with whom we spoke had grown up in poverty, and many had come from disorganized and strife-ridden families in which the major role models did not by example communicate the value of education and self-empowerment. When we ended the ethnography, we shared some of the demoralization that pervaded the lives of so many of the families we studied. The barriers they faced in their attempts even to get by, let alone move out of poverty and into self-sufficiency, were daunting, and it was clear that many of those barriers were formal parts of the social insurance systems upon which they depended. We asked ourselves how we might improve the system so that it empowers individuals and families to succeed and to escape the physical and psychological damage that life at the margin can cause. In Chapter 8, we offer our suggestions.

8

Health Care for All Americans

The health care financing crisis that threatens the health and well-being of the poor families whose story we have told in these chapters is part of a far more serious problem of equity, fairness, and access to social services that affects the health of our nation in various domains. The poor not only are exposed to serious physical and mental health risks but also forced to rely on a system of care that is fragmented and often inadequate. This vulnerability is clearly associated with the low productivity and low earnings capacities of individuals with little education and few job skills. Those individual vulnerabilities, however, are not just the result of poor personal decisions; they result in large part from the restricted opportunities available to those who grow up in low-resource barrios and ghettos. Low education and limited job skills are also the result of the threats to health to which those growing up in such circumstances are exposed. A rather large body of research, in addition to our study, documents the clear association between the lack of health insurance coverage, inadequate health care, and poor health outcomes (Institute of Medicine 2001; Institute of Medicine 2002a). It is clear as well that incomplete health care coverage of the population incurs substantial social costs (Institute of Medicine 2003a; Institute of Medicine 2003b).

The previous chapters have illustrated the importance of Medicaid and SCHIP to pregnant women and families with children. Medicaid has also become the payer of last resort for elderly and disabled adults who have exhausted their resources and cannot pay for acute or long-term care. Despite the fact that a large portion of every state's Medicaid budget is provided by the federal government, states are facing an ever-growing burden that will only increase as the baby-boom generation begins to need care for the diseases of aging. As a result, states have implemented a number of mechanisms for reducing, or at least slowing, the growth of their Medicaid programs (Smith et al. 2004). These include restrictions on enrollment, reductions in services, and limits on the number of prescription drugs covered by Medicaid (Cunningham 2005; Morden and Sullivan 2005).

This crisis in Medicaid places families like those in our study at serious risk of further erosion of their health care coverage. If balancing state budgets requires reductions in Medicaid, poor working-age families with children will no doubt be among the most seriously affected. Although nearly three-quarters of Medicaid participants are children in poor families, over three-quarters of Medicaid revenues go to pay for the long-term care of the elderly and disabled (Liska 1997). As the population ages and as the number of older individuals in need of long-term care grows, the pressure to cut program costs may fall heaviest on children and poor working-age families.

Even when they had no coverage for themselves, our respondents persevered in their attempts to get and keep health care and other services for their children. The complexity of the eligibility rules and the practical difficulties that arose in dealing with often contradictory and confusing bureaucracies meant that they were not always successful in getting care for their children. Although coverage from Medicaid for infants and young children in very poor families is readily available, coverage for older children – especially, as we showed in the last chapter, in families close to 200 percent of poverty – is more difficult to obtain, and even when a parent manages to obtain coverage for their older children, that coverage is easily lost.

Since the time of the initial survey and the beginning of the ethnography, certain reforms to the application process for Medicaid, including such conveniences as mail-in applications and less frequent and easier recertification procedures, promised to improve the situation somewhat, and SCHIP, which was not yet in operation in Texas when the study began, has also improved the situation for children in families with incomes above the federal poverty line. However, even though the program has been very successful in enrolling children, as we write this book, Texas has already cut back on its SCHIP program, and children are losing their coverage (Dunkelberg and O'Malley 2004). As our ethnographic interviews revealed, problems of access and continuity of coverage are still common, and they are not likely to be eliminated as long as we rely on a two-tiered system with shrinking employment-based coverage for the middle class and the stigmatizing means-tested safety net approach for the poor. Furthermore, low-income workers will continue to be caught in situations without employer-sponsored health insurance while remaining ineligible for public health coverage programs. The most glaring failure of this system is its implicit inability to provide coverage to working poor families and to nonelderly adults.

Medicaid and SCHIP: Successes and Failures

In the absence of universal health care coverage or a single-payer system, Medicaid represents the cornerstone of the means-tested health care safety net for both the young and their families. Medicaid provides coverage for infants and young children, as well as for the low-income disabled and those over sixty-five who need long-term care. Yet both Medicaid and private health insurance coverage for children have been on the decline since the passage of the 1996 welfare reform act (Chavkin, Romero, and Wise 2000; Committee on Child Health Financing 2001; Ku and Bruen 2000; Rowland, Salganicoff, and Keenan 1999). This decline occurred even though since 2000 federal spending on Medicaid has increased nearly 9 percent per year, largely offsetting declines in employer-based coverage for children (Holahan and Bruen 2003). Even with the increase in Medicaid expenditures, however, nearly 11 percent of all children (8.2 million) lacked health insurance coverage in 2002 (Kohn, Hasty, and Henderson 2002) even though more than half were eligible for public health coverage (Starfield 2000).

Despite its objective of increasing coverage among working poor families, SCHIP has had only a modest impact on the health insurance crisis among children (Chavkin, Romero, and Wise 2000; Kohn, Hasty, and Henderson 2002; Weinick and Krauss 2000; Zuckerman et al. 2001). As a joint federal/state program, it inevitably responds to state budgetary pressures. Even as states stand to lose important federal matching funds, states such as Texas have reduced Medicaid and SCHIP spending. The experience with this program reveals again the limits of a means-tested approach to health care coverage for the unemployed and working poor.

To summarize the two major components of the health care crisis among children consist of the large number of children in families that earn too much to qualify for Medicaid or SCHIP and high levels of nonparticipation even among income-eligible children (Ku and Bruen 1999; Salsberry 2003). Many explanations have been offered for low rates of Medicaid coverage and for the decline in Medicaid coverage after the 1996 welfare reform legislation. The most common explanations focus on specific access barriers, such as complicated administrative procedures that discourage those who qualify from seeking assistance (Boslaugh et al. 1999; Chavkin and Wise 2002; Kohn, Hasty, and Henderson 2002; Salsberry 2003; Vastag 2002). Among our heavily Hispanic sample, language barriers and the stigma associated with public assistance also contribute to lowered participation rates (Flores et al. 1998; Perloff 1999; Thamer and Richard 1997; Weinick and Krauss 2000). Many other factors no doubt contribute to the failure of public programs to reach eligible families in need.

What remains indisputable is that the lack of health care coverage among the poor has potentially serious long-term consequences because it is associated with inadequate preventive care and a heightened probability of serious childhood illnesses (Adler and Newman 2002; Davidoff et al. 2000; Institute of Medicine 2001; Institute of Medicine 2002a; Rowland, Salganicoff, and Keenan 1999; Schur and Albers 1995; Starfield 2000). Health conditions that interfere with social and emotional development can undermine future productivity and increase the risk of intergenerational poverty (MacLanahan and Sandefur 1994). The risk of lowered productivity among children who will make up the labor force of the future places the nation in long-term jeopardy.

Sources of Vulnerability among Our Ethnographic Families

At the time we were recruiting our families into the ethnographic study, all three states had their own set of policies related to the implementation of the federal law and the extent to which they offered medical coverage beyond what was required. Of the three states, Texas had perhaps the least inclusive policies for covering children in low-income families because the state only expanded eligibility beyond the minimum federal requirements in a few areas, including care for very young children and the creation of some programs that offered "transitional" benefits to mothers and children leaving welfare. These families could receive such benefits for between four and twelve months. However, the regulations by which Texas measured eligibility and certified families continued to create considerable difficulties in two areas: (1) the income guidelines by which low-income, non-TANF families were eligible for Medicaid, and (2) the programs through which families could secure and keep transitional programs when they left welfare.

The eligibility determination process was complicated in all three cities. Families had to bring documentation related to income, child well-being, and the father's capacity to support the child to the welfare office. Mothers who misunderstood the process or failed to provide required documentation often found that one or more family members were dropped from TANF or denied Medicaid. Families had to inform welfare offices when they moved, when they changed jobs, when they earned or received extra income as a gift, when they had someone else staying with them, or when they sent a child to live somewhere else. In the initial planning stages of the study, we considered offering the families a small honorarium as a motivation to participate and to compensate them for the fairly time-intensive task we were asking of them. However, we quickly found out that a gift of even a small amount of money would have to be reported to the welfare office as income, and we decided to give the families gift certificates and other noncash rewards in order not to violate the formal requirements.

Many families did not understand that transitional benefits were available and that being dropped from the TANF rolls did not automatically mean the loss of Medicaid eligibility. Because certification for Medicaid was based on the same application forms as the application for TANF, and because eligibility for Medicaid and TANF was determined at the same office, many families believed they were linked and that the loss of TANF eligibility also meant the loss of Medicaid eligibility. Other families found the reapplication process for Medicaid after they left the TANF rolls to be overwhelmingly complicated. Indeed, we encountered three different pathways to Medicaid transitional benefits, each of which required somewhat different applications at different times. We were never certain of the exact requirements, and we suspect that many of the caseworkers who were providing information to our families were not either. It is hardly surprising that many poor families found the system impenetrable. Of course, as we mentioned, many of these barriers have been addressed by legislation that has streamlined the application and recertification processes. Nonetheless, given the requirement that one establish need and periodically recertify, serious barriers to continuous and full coverage remain.

Taxation and the Public Weal

Since at least the Reagan administration, supply-side economics has come to mean an almost exclusive concern with tax cuts under the assumption that reductions in taxes directly increase investment and productivity in ways that will eventually offset the more serious negative consequences of social service reductions for subgroups of the population. In addition, since the Reagan administration, public policy has focused on minimizing the role of the federal government in social services, and rather than focusing on ensuring national optimal levels of health, our public agenda has moved toward the devolution of federal functions to the states, where budget-strapped legislatures are frequently forced to reduce public health and medical care funding. Even in this climate of reduced federal control over social welfare policy, however, the importance of health and the plight of the working poor have led Congress to mandate extensions of coverage to children in families above the federal poverty line.

For the more advanced welfare states of Europe, health care is viewed as a central component of a system that seeks to optimize the quality of the labor force. From this perspective, workers are not simply interchangeable and easily replaceable inputs into some production process; rather, they are citizens and human beings whose lives must be rich and productive if they are to contribute to the economy and to civil society more generally. Such an approach focuses on the vital importance of investments in people, including their health and education, rather than on tax cuts alone. Although even the advanced welfare states must face the realities of fiscal limitations, they are far less concerned with minimizing governmental functions than with ensuring adequate social investment. This focus stems from the assumption that in order for a society to function well and for individuals to thrive and contribute to economic productivity, they must partake of all of the rights of citizenship, including adequate material welfare.

There are clearly times when reductions in marginal tax rates are a good idea, and there are many government-supported programs that are in serious need of reform and increased efficiency. Yet the basic fact remains that the basis of economic productivity, especially in an increasingly information-dominated world, depends on a healthy, vital, and educated workforce. Unfortunately, as we have shown, the systems for assuring the health of the workforce are in disarray, a term employed in a report by the Institute of Medicine of the National Academy of Sciences to describe our public health system (Committee on Assuring the Health of the Public in the 21st Century 2002). The unemployed and the working poor are not only handicapped in their ability to get the preventive and acute health care they need but are also at high risk of compromised health as the result of fundamental shortcomings in our public health system. As the data we have presented clearly show, these are particularly serious problems for African Americans and Hispanics.

Although modern medical care has clearly contributed to both the increased length and higher quality of our lives, basic public health measures, such as ensuring clean water and safe food, developing safe workplaces, providing family planning, and especially the delivery of childhood immunization, have played a major role in increasing life spans (Centers for Disease Control 1999). Yet, as important as immunizations are in preventing childhood illnesses, many children are not fully immunized. Again, African American and Hispanic children are at the greatest risk of incomplete immunization. Between 1996 and 2001, the immunization gap between non-Hispanic white, African American, and Hispanic children widened. In 2001, approximately one-quarter of African American and Hispanic children were incompletely immunized (Chu, Barker, and Smith 2004). This fact adds to the already elevated risk profile associated with poverty and threatens the quality of life of millions of young Americans and the future productivity of the labor force (Angel and Angel 1993). In addition to lower immunization rates, African American and Hispanic children fare badly in terms of other basic public health measures. For instance, although the proportion of children who are overweight has increased among all groups, the increase has been particularly pronounced among black and Hispanic children (Hedley et al. 2004; Hoelscher et al. 2004; Ogden et al. 2002). These children are at elevated risk of the early onset of all of the negative consequences of obesity.

In addition to the crisis in health care coverage, it is therefore imperative that we recognize the public health care crisis of the poor as a collective problem that affects each of us directly. Ultimately, education, nutrition, immunization, safe neighborhoods, secure families, and the rest of what makes for a happy and healthy childhood and adulthood are as important as preventive and acute medical care in improving lives. As we have argued, the health of the public is a central policy concern because our collective well-being is made up of the aggregate well-being of individuals and depends directly upon a healthy workforce. In 1945, there were slightly over forty workers for each retiree; by 2003, there were slightly more than three workers supporting each retired American (Social Security Administration 2004a; Social Security Administration 2004b). In the future, the number of workers supporting each retiree will decline even further, and if Social Security remains a pay-as-you-go system in which the support of the retired population comes directly from the paychecks of those who are still working, those workers will have to contribute a larger fraction of their income in Social Security and Medicare taxes (Bongaarts 2004). A highly productive workforce that will be willing and able to bear the burden requires investment and nurturing. With inadequate investments in the health and education of people, or inadequate investments in major segments of the population, even a dynamic and powerful nation like ours could well see its global dominance erode.

Realistic Options for Insuring Everyone

Universal health care coverage has never even come close to passage in the United States. The most recent attempt, during the early years of the Clinton administration, clearly demonstrated the obstacles. President Clinton and many other observers imagined that the time for comprehensive coverage had finally arrived, and initially the proposal seemed to have broad support (Skocpol 1996; Starr 1994). Unfortunately, that support turned out to be much thinner than the proponents of universal coverage had hoped, and opposition by segments of the insurance and medical establishments, in combination with serious political blunders by the Clinton administration itself, resulted in a resounding defeat that carried over into losses for the Democratic Party in the 1994 midterm elections (Daniels, Light, and Caplan 1996; Skocpol 1996). That experience, in combination with earlier failures at fundamental reform, might well lead one to despair of the possibility of ever introducing universal health care coverage in the United States.

As we have noted throughout our discussion, however, there is reason to believe that the forces that impelled the Clinton administration to attempt radical rather than piecemeal reform will in the not too distant future again move us in the direction of a more universal and coordinated system of health care financing and delivery. The aging of the population, in addition to medical progress and apparently unending health care inflation, will eventually require some greater central coordination and control. Unfortunately, it will also require some form of rationing. In their current forms, market mechanisms and public program extensions alone will never both ensure universal health care coverage and allow the nation to control inflationary health care costs. In this chapter, we relate what we discovered in our study to the health reform proposals that have been offered in recent years. Our conclusion is that comprehensive and universal coverage cannot be achieved through piecemeal reform or the extension of current programs alone unless that extension is motivated by the ultimate objective of universal coverage. By now there appears to be a fairly general consensus that a substantial fraction of the more than forty million uninsured Americans can only be covered by a publicly funded safety net. The only debate relates to the extent and generosity of that safety net and how it can be financed and administered in a way that will make it sustainable in the long run.

Given the political and economic realities of the U.S. health care marketplace, it is unrealistic to imagine that a single-payer system is possible in the short term. Proposals that ignore the interests of the health insurance industry or the market forces that govern the medical marketplace, as the Clinton plan did, are doomed to failure and do not represent useful contributions to the reform debate. New initiatives based on public–private partnerships (PPPs) and other organizational and financing innovations will no doubt be tried, and some will prove effective in bringing some of the currently uninsured into the system (Rosenau 2000; Sparer 2000). The increasing reliance of Medicaid on private managed-care plans is one example of such public–private ventures (Sparer 2000). If such initiatives result in near-universal coverage for basic preventive as well as acute and catastrophic care, progress toward the objectives of a universal health care system will have been made. The efficiency of the system that emerges will have to be assessed in practice and the determination and implementation of best-practice models made at multiple levels of government and the health care delivery system.

One of the major roadblocks to the adoption of universal health care coverage in the United States has been our federated system, in which states retain a large part of the control over social service delivery. In addition to obstacles to change, however, that system also provides us with unique opportunities to experiment. In effect, we can conduct a fifty-state experiment in how to define best practices and how to provide services to the currently uninsured. Today, states learn from one another concerning the best way to provide public health care. Again, the experience of the Clinton administration with radical reform and our current political climate make it clear that we will have to look to the states for innovations, at least in the short term. Even in the long term, the fundamental state-based nature of the American political system will have to be taken into account.

In all likelihood, a realistic comprehensive system will consist of an expanded and subsidized employment-based system accompanied by an expanded safety net. Only experimentation will eventually reveal which specific approach is both equitable and economically efficient. A health care system that consumes an ever-growing share of gross domestic product (GDP) is, by definition, unsustainable. A universal health care system with strong central controls will have far more possibilities for cost control and equitable rationing than less coordinated and more decentralized approaches. Such a system, however, will in all likelihood be very different from the one that has evolved over the last century, and it would be hard to implement in our currently highly privatized and decentralized medical marketplace. Our study, however, clearly reveals the pitfalls and problems faced by families without dependable health insurance. Families are best served by coverage that is continuous and seamless and in which the lapses in coverage and the incomplete nature of coverage, both for older children and adults, are eliminated. Such a system will inevitably be very different from the one with which we are familiar.

The Major Barriers to Change

In the previous chapters, we have outlined the major obstacles to fundamental change in the U.S. health care financing system. There are, of course, many such obstacles, and before we proceed to an examination of the major proposals for reform of the health care delivery system it would be useful to remind ourselves of the basic barriers to change that have undermined all previous attempts at major restructuring of the health care financing system. Put most simply, the major barrier to any attempt at reform of the current system has been its fundamental compatibility with the interests of almost everyone involved, including business, labor, middle-class employees, insurers, the health care industry, and even government. Multiple and powerful interests support the status quo and, at most, favor small-scale and incremental changes that do not threaten the basic market basis of the health care industry. In addition, the fact that those who are left out of the current system lack the economic or political power to further their interests ensures that there is no organized opposition.

Of course, the stability of the status quo also reflects the real success of the current system in covering the majority of the population. The fact that the vast majority of Americans are insured by either employer-sponsored private health plans or one of several public programs works against change (Hacker 2002; Starr 1982). Most people draw on different health care plans over the course of their lives, and most remain almost continuously covered, at least for basic care. Middle-class individuals who have employer-sponsored group health insurance that provides comprehensive family coverage at a reasonable cost correctly assume that they would lose some of those benefits and that they would have to pay more for them under any proposal for covering the uninsured. Despite the efficiencies that any new system might introduce, it is highly unlikely that the uninsured could be covered on a cost-neutral basis. Total costs would probably increase substantially, even as those individuals who currently have comprehensive coverage are required to pay more for less. Those over the age of sixty-five and their representatives, such as the American Association of Retired Persons (AARP), are less concerned with universal coverage for the entire population than they are with issues that affect the elderly, such as prescription drug coverage under Medicare.

Yet it is increasingly obvious that it is impossible to ignore the serious shortcomings of the present system. Although it provides the world's best medicine to insured middle-class families, the failure of the private insurance/public safety net alternative upon which we have relied since the 1960s provides strong evidence that the current system simply cannot cover everyone without major reform. Despite the fact that the United States devotes a far larger share of GDP to health care than other nations, the system is seriously incomplete in terms of coverage of the population. As a result of the factors we have discussed in the preceding chapters, including the rising cost to employers, the number of uninsured Americans is projected to increase (Gilmer and Kronick 2005). Even if they retain their employer-sponsored coverage, more Americans will find that they are underinsured and do not have access to the full range of care they need at the same time that they will have to pay more for the care they receive (Schoen et al. 2004). For the working poor, work never has been a route to insurance adequacy. At the bottom of the job distribution, going to work can mean losing one's insurance coverage (Holl, Slack, and Stevens 2005). As we have shown in our ethnographic case studies, the health care safety net is far from seamless or comprehensive, and the lives of families who must rely on it are disrupted by uncertainty and instability. As the previous chapters have shown, the incomplete and inadequate nature of the safety net itself contributes significantly to that instability and uncertainty and the difficulty many families face in improving their lot.

The Range of Solutions: Proposals for Reform

Although medicine is clearly a business, economists have long pointed out that market principles do not readily apply to health care. In a classic article published over four decades ago, Nobel Prize–winning economist Kenneth Arrow explained why basic competitive market principles do not apply to the health care industry (Arrow 1963). Arrow argued that unlike food or clothing, for which demand is steady and continuous, the demand for health care is irregular and unpredictable.

Arrow presented a very complex argument in which he made the case for the special nature of health care as an item of consumption. Some elements of health care certainly fit this model, especially at the time Arrow presented the argument. Perhaps it is time to think of health care in a different way, however, given advances in medical care and the role of medicine in health maintenance as well as the treatment of disease. Today, routine health care is not all that different from other predictable expenditures. Obviously, the need for extraordinary or heroic treatment for rare conditions is unpredictable but it is clear from our interviews that the need for routine care is not. That routine care is not a budgetable expense for poor families, not because it is unpredictable but because on a limited income they simply cannot afford it.

During the twentieth century, medicine evolved from a body of knowledge and practice that was inexpensive and ineffective to a system of scientifically based knowledge and interventions that is highly effective and necessary for the highest levels of physical and mental functioning. It is also, however, hugely expensive. All but the most routine and minor care is too expensive to be dealt with in the ordinary low-income or even middle-income family budget. Indeed, medical care today might usefully be compared to education, for which the concept of "insurance" is clearly inappropriate. One does not "insure" one's children against the need for education. Literacy is such a core component of a productive life that in all developed societies the state treats basic education, at least in principle, as a collective good provided at public expense.

It would probably be useful to drop the term "insurance" from discussions of health care financing in general. Some radical proposals would eliminate the insurance industry as well as the insurance principle (Bodenheimer 1990). One of the major problems with a system based on insurance principles and the private market is the need on the part of the insurer to exclude those in greatest need of services. In order to make a profit, insurance companies are forced to "underwrite," a term that refers to the exclusion of "adverse risks," or individuals who are sick or likely to become so (Aaron 1991; Fein 1986; Light 1992). By its very nature, such a system cannot be inclusive or universal. As the populations of the developed nations age, and as public health and medicine become more effective at treating illness, even serious chronic diseases such as cancer and heart disease become more prevalent because individuals afflicted with them survive longer. In any human population, the benefits of a long life are inevitably accompanied by the diseases of aging. Effective medicine is increasingly a double-edged sword. We will all eventually need significant amounts of medical care, and in the future our society will have to develop equitable ways of rationing that care.

Even with Medicare, many elderly individuals pay a large fraction of their incomes for health care (Moon 1996). Low-income families deal with unstable health care coverage, medical debt, and often forgo treatment. Ours is a system in which the rationing of health care is based on the ability to pay, which seriously penalizes our study families and, increasingly, segments of the working class. Our study has led us to propose that we begin thinking of health as a social good, the production of which is a collective responsibility, just like the education of our children. The old are our parents and ourselves in the future, and children are our only hope for that future. Their health and productivity are among our most precious resources. Anything short of complete and continuous health care coverage, as well as a serious commitment to the universality of public health, is shortsighted. Readily available health care is an important building block in constructing future economic and social well-being.

In our opinion, the United States, like every other developed nation in the world, should provide some level of comprehensive health care to all citizens. A society's level of concern for the health of its citizens reflects basic values and its sense of community. In health, as in education, it is in the interests of the larger society to make sure that the largest possible proportion of the population gets adequate services. Given that premise, the problem of how to implement it remains. Of all of the alternatives that have been discussed since the Truman administration, a single-payer, comprehensive system of health care coverage most nearly satisfies that objective. As part of our conclusion, it would be useful to examine the general mechanisms that have been proposed in the name of health care financing reforms. Rather than referring to specific legislators or specific bills, most of which will be replaced or extended by other proposals in the relatively short term, we present the general characteristics of the major proposals that come up time and again in various forms and we discuss their strengths and weaknesses. Our discussion parallels closely that presented by the Institute of Medicine in its 2004 recommendations for fundamental health care financing reform (Institute of Medicine 2004).

Basic Requirements for an Equitable and Sustainable Health Care System

There appears to be fairly wide consensus on the characteristics of an equitable and efficient health care system. The dilemma, of course, is how to establish such an ideal system that is both politically and economically feasible. In an ideal system, health care coverage should be universal, continuous, and affordable for individuals and families. Access to adequate health care should not be limited by means tests, age, current health condition, or any other individual characteristic. Both treatment and preventive measures should be included because they are essential aspects of a complete system of health care. Currently, public programs pay insufficient attention to prevention and to public health.

In order to ensure the greatest possible degree of continuity of care, there should be as few transfers as possible from one health care delivery system to another. Currently, even families that manage to maintain fairly continuous health coverage are often forced to switch from one provider and one health care system to another as they move between welfare and work and between jobs. Each of these changes can mean that the health care coverage for different members of the family varies greatly even over short periods. The requirement of affordability is, of course, central both for families and their employers. As many employers, and particularly small businesses, find themselves faced with rapidly rising health insurance costs, many are dropping their plans, and those that retain them have no choice but to pass an increasing proportion of the costs of coverage on to their employees in the form of higher premiums, co-payments, and deductibles. For many working poor families, the requirement of affordability is simply not met. Because their employers cannot provide the coverage that low-wage working families need, publicly funded care is essential in order to ensure an equitable system. Unfortunately, as we have shown, the current multiprogram public system is incapable of meeting the basic standards of equity and efficiency.

Of course, affordability is not only a concern for individuals and employers but a central concern for society at large. Any reformed health care system that would cover all Americans must be sustainable in the long run, which means that it must be economically efficient as well as equitable. Currently, medical inflation is growing at a rate that each year consumes a larger fraction of GDP. The expansion of coverage to those who are currently inadequately insured must be accompanied by cost-containment efforts that may make such reforms unpopular. Bringing more than forty million uninsured individuals into the system will not be cost-neutral even with substantial efficiencies and savings. From society's perspective, therefore, any viable health insurance scheme must be affordable, as well as manageable and efficient, and it should be designed to enhance the well-being and productivity of the population at large.

The possibilities for reform of our current health care financing system range from maintaining the status quo to the adoption of a completely universal and comprehensive single-payer system in which the federal government assumes primary responsibility for the health care needs of all citizens. Between these two extremes lie many possibilities that combine proposals for expanding existing public systems such as Medicare and Medicaid, tax credits to employers and employees, employer mandates in which employers would be required to provide coverage, perhaps with public subsidies, and individual mandates in which employees and those not in the labor force would be required to participate in available health plans, again with incentives or financial support. Many useful overviews are available (e.g., Altman, Reinhardt, and Shields 1998; Institute of Medicine, 2004). Many of these proposals are based upon the expansion of health care consumer purchasing cooperatives, which were a prominent part of the Clinton plan, in which the pooling of purchasing power increases the leverage of individuals and small businesses.

Each of these intermediate proposals would probably increase the number of insured Americans, but unless they included universal mandates they would not cover everyone, and as health care costs increase, the number of families covered and the amount and quality of health care they receive might well drop. Those who will benefit least from most of the proposed reforms are individuals in families like those in our study. In addition to failing to offer comprehensive and universal coverage, the proposals for highly complicated combined systems that include employer and employee tax credits, mandates for both groups, and expansions of public coverage may well introduce administrative costs that could add to medical cost inflation. They could also create unequal categories of coverage and be based on eligibility criteria that continue to leave large groups of people uninsured. As is the case with our current system, African Americans and Hispanics would probably be the big losers.

In the following discussion, we will not focus on the details of the relative cost of the proposals that have been offered. Such assessments are based on complex models with many and profound assumptions that may or may not be justified. In any case, the specifics of cost and efficiency calculations will take decades of experimentation and trial and error. In what follows, we discuss the shortcomings of each of these proposed mechanisms for expanding health care coverage in terms of the extent to which they might reasonably be expected to address the needs of the sorts of poor families we studied. Our objective is to begin a debate about the potential for extending health coverage universally in a continuous and affordable manner.

Conflicting Objectives

The debate over specific health care system reforms in the United States has been influenced by several contradictory objectives. First, the desire to extend coverage to the uninsured conflicts with the need to contain medical care costs. Administratively, the desire to maintain the state's role in regulating public health care programs conflicts with the need for national-level coordination. From the point of view of current insurers, the desire to preserve the rights of insurers to define their own products and to preserve the rights of employers to offer coverage or not conflicts with the need to ensure high-quality coverage and require employers to offer coverage or pay into state-sponsored plans. These conflicting objectives reflect both practical administrative problems and difficulties that arise from the desire to preserve the market and employment basis of health insurance in the United States. Any future health care system reform will have to take this complex set of conflicting objectives into account if it is to be politically viable and economically realistic.

Since the 1980s, significant health care financing reforms have been passed by Congress. The most important of these have extended coverage for specific groups of the uninsured or underinsured, including the low-income elderly, the disabled, and children in families with incomes below 200 percent of the federal poverty line (FPL). Unfortunately, these health care financing reforms have failed to reduce the overall number of uninsured Americans and, in fact, that number has continued to increase along with the size of the population (Institute of Medicine 2004; Mills and Bhandari 2003). During the 1980s and 1990s, eligibility for Medicaid and the State Children's Health Insurance Program (SCHIP) was extended to nearly all children in families with incomes below 200 percent of the FPL (Broaddus and Ku 2000). Yet many children do not participate, and fully half of those children who remain uninsured qualify for these programs but are not enrolled (Dubay, Haley, and Kenney 2002; Kenney, Haley, and Tebay 2003). In addition to eligible children who are not enrolled, these reforms have left many poor elderly individuals, including a large fraction of minority Americans, vulnerable to crushing medical debt. As we noted earlier, even with Medicare, the elderly spend a large fraction of their limited incomes on health care, and many face impoverishment when they must use long term care (Angel and Angel 1997).

For preretirement-age adults, federal efforts have focused on improving aspects of employment-based insurance through such legislation as the Consolidated Omnibus Budget Reconciliation Act (COBRA) of 1985 and the Health Insurance Portability and Accountability Act (HIPAA) of 1996. This legislation provides for the portability of insurance from one employer to another and allows individuals to remain in an employer's group health plan at his or her own expense for at least a while after the termination of his or her employment. In addition, the Trade Act (TA) of 2002 provides assistance for individuals who have lost their jobs as the result of international competition (Institute of Medicine 2004). At the same time that federal law attempts to preserve coverage for those who have employer-sponsored plans, another aspect of the law, specifically in the form of the Employee Retirement and Income Security Act (ERISA) of 1974, has limited states' ability to mandate coverage for employees (Butler 2000a; Butler 2000b; National Association of Insurance Commissioners 1999).

Despite the government's piecemeal efforts to retain coverage for the nonwelfare unemployed, the basic problem remains that if one loses one's job and does not find another one quickly, one's group insurance premiums eventually become unaffordable. Although there can be no doubt that portability and continuity of coverage are desirable, if that portability and continuity depend on the continuity of employment, periods of unemployment will almost inevitably translate into the loss of insurance for many individuals, especially the long-term unemployed. The result is that few mechanisms currently exist for dealing with the problem of the lack of insurance for the long-term unemployed or for those workers in jobs that do not offer work continuity or coverage.

Realistic Options for Reform

Since President Truman's unsuccessful attempt to pass the Wagner-Murray-Dingell bill during the 1940s, most proposals for health care financing reform, with the exception of President Clinton's failed plan, have been incremental (Maioni 1998; Marmor 1973; Marmor and Barer 1997; Starr 1982). As we have explained, no substantial constituency for radical reform has ever emerged in the United States, largely because of the success of our employment-based system in covering the majority of middle-class families. By the 1950s, private Blue Cross/Blue Shield plans were the dominant form of coverage in the nation and our current employer-based system was firmly entrenched (Cunningham and Cunningham 1997; Starr 1982). The passage of Medicare and Medicaid legislation addressed some of the most glaring shortcomings of the purely market-based system (Fox 1986; Hacker 1997; Schlesinger and Kronebusch 1990). Even the perceived financial crisis that has accompanied the growth of medical costs has not resulted in serious broad-based support for attempts to bring about radical reform (Kahn and Pollack 2001).

Although cost containment and efficiency must be central objectives of any reform, from our perspective universal and comprehensive coverage is imperative and justifiable on the basis of principle alone. Our individual and collective welfare depends on providing the full range of social citizenship rights outlined by T. H. Marshall with which we began this study (Marshall 1950). Incremental reforms that fail to achieve universality and comprehensiveness are unacceptable because they are inequitable, unjust, and economically short-sighted (Himmelstein and Woolhandler 2003; Weil 2001). Incremental reforms that eventually arrive at universal and comprehensive coverage are far more logical and should define our longer-term objectives.

Many potential reforms of our current system have been offered. Some, such as medical savings accounts, are simply traditional insurance policies with a high deductible combined with a plan that allows individuals to save pretax dollars to pay the high deductibles. These plans cost less because they only pay for major medical expenses after one has paid the deductible of $1,500 or more from the savings account. Such plans are popular with conservatives because they largely reaffirm the status quo (Robinson 2004). Although medical savings accounts are becoming quite popular among the middle class because they allow a family to set aside pretax dollars that can be accumulated from year to year if they are not used, such plans are irrelevant to families with limited resources such as those in our study. They benefit those in the highest tax brackets, for whom pretax savings are a real benefit. The tax advantages are far less valuable to those in lower tax brackets and of no use at all to families that have no income to save or any tax liability. As we saw for those receiving public benefits, any savings at all reduces those benefits, so plans based on savings do not speak to the needs of the poor.

Other reforms that retain the basic components of the current system without simply reaffirming the status quo include proposals to extend existing programs such as Medicaid, SCHIP, and Medicare to include a larger fraction of the working poor, the unemployed, and adults younger than sixty-five who do not have insurance (Davis and Schoen 2003; Davis, Schoen, and Schoenbaum 2000; Feder et al. 2001). These proposals and others often include a federal tax credit that would allow individuals to buy insurance through their employer or some other group or private provider at an affordable cost. Those individuals and families with very low incomes who incur no tax obligation would receive what is essentially a subsidy with which they could purchase coverage (Davis and Schoen 2003; Feder et al. 2001; Institute of Medicine 2004; Pauly and Herring 2001).

Under such plans, Medicaid and SCHIP could be merged into a joint federal/state program and Medicare eligibility would be lowered to age fifty-five, an age at which an individual could buy into the system by paying a small premium. One important characteristic of such proposals for expanding existing programs is that they do not alter the current employment-based system and are not mandatory. Like the current safety net approach, they would retain the current two-tiered system in which those with employer-sponsored coverage have a different and usually better set of choices than those with publicly funded coverage. Under such proposals, tax incentives for employers and employees would remain unchanged and individuals could participate or not depending on whether they wished to avail themselves of the tax credit. One benefit is that these proposals build upon existing administrative structures and experiences. On the other hand, they retain most of the shortcomings of the current system in which families that are eligible simply do not participate. They would not, therefore, result in universal and comprehensive coverage because they reaffirm the two-tiered approach for the middle class and the poor.

More radical proposals would require employers to provide coverage to their employees and also require employees to accept that coverage (Institute of Medicine 2004; Wicks 2003). Voluntary systems create a "free rider" problem because those without insurance receive subsidized medical care when they fall ill (Goodman 2001). That care must be paid for by someone, and the burden usually falls upon the insured population or the taxpayer. Massachusetts and Hawaii have experimented with such systems (Himmelstein and Woolhandler 2003). Because small employers cannot afford to provide coverage and their employees cannot afford the premiums, subsidies to employers and an expanded public safety net based on Medicaid and SCHIP or some other program would be necessary (Institute of Medicine 2004). Many of these proposals include the development of large purchaser pools so that small employers and individuals could join together and have the same ability to negotiate with insurers and health care providers as large companies (Curtis, Neuschler, and Forland 2001). Despite many potential problems, including deciding who would negotiate for the group, because of the mandated nature of coverage such proposals would come closer to universal coverage. Proposals that focus solely on employers and employees, however, do not address the needs of the unemployed, the temporarily employed, or those employed part-time.

Other proposals that focus on individuals and families rather than on employees propose a subsidy to individuals for the purpose of purchasing health care coverage from a range of choices. The key aspect of such proposals is that individuals would be required to purchase at least a basic plan for themselves and their dependents (Institute of Medicine 2004). The subsidy that families would receive, which could be used only for purchasing health coverage and would be based on family size and income, would be paid as a tax credit that could be used before the end of the tax year or as a subsidy for those with no tax liability. This approach would take the government into new territory in terms of administration and would result in the elimination of the current employer and employee tax credit and the elimination of Medicaid and SCHIP because they would be redundant. The mandatory nature of coverage would require mechanisms, perhaps tied to income tax collection, for assuring that individuals have purchased the required minimal coverage. These proposals clearly come far closer to covering everyone than those that stay closer to the status quo.

The final, and most radical, approach would be a single-payer system in which the federal government would assure comprehensive coverage for all citizens (Himmelstein and Woolhandler 2003; Institute of Medicine 2004). This path would require a new federal agency, perhaps with regional offices in each state, that would set coverage standards and deal with providers of all sorts from doctors to pharmacies to hospitals and long-term care facilities. This agency would review claims and process payments much as Medicaid does now (Institute of Medicine 2004). The package of services offered would have to be decided upon based on sound economic and clinical criteria, but it would cover both preventive and acute care for all citizens. The program would almost inevitably include options for supplemental coverage for services that are not part of the basic plan. Those who use services might be required to pay a small co-payment at the point of service, although some proposals reject any out-of-pocket payment as a barrier to access (Himmelstein and Woolhandler 2003).

A single-payer system would be funded through a national budget within which cost containment could be more efficiently achieved. Some proponents believe that the savings that could be achieved through the elimination of duplicate services and excessive administrative costs would make such a plan almost cost-neutral (Himmelstein and Woolhandler 2003). Such claims are probably too optimistic because even with substantial savings in terms of efficiency, bringing more than forty million uninsured Americans, basically the same number that receive Social Security, into the system will inevitably incur new costs. Many of these uninsured individuals have serious medical care needs that have gone untreated. Clearly, a fully comprehensive and universal health care system would represent a radical departure from our current complex private insurance system, and that fact remains one of the major roadblocks to the adoption of such a system.

Many critics and even supporters of universal coverage believe that a fully public single-payer system is politically unrealistic in the United States (Tooker 2002). Individuals and organizations who profit directly from the current market-based system are unlikely to welcome major reforms that affect their economic interests, and they have powerful political allies. Aside from those with direct financial interests in the status quo, additional opposition to universal health insurance arises from Americans' distrust of big government. Some observers simply do not believe that government can achieve equitable and just ends without distorting the system or introducing a stultifying bureaucracy. It is unlikely that a radical shift to a single-payer universal system will occur quickly, and the more realistic option is a comprehensive system that is based on a mix of mechanisms that functionally achieve universal coverage (Bodenheimer 2003).

As we stated, the technical aspects of the health care financing system that finally prevails lie beyond the scope of our discussion. As the history of health care financing in the United States attests, much of what emerges represents the unintended consequences of incremental developments rather than the result of deliberate public policy. The political reality is that decisions that are made during one period create institutions and expectations that resist change even when change is called for. Welfare began in the 1930s as a small program within the Social Security bill to provide support to widows. Over the years, it evolved into something quite different in response to forces that the framers never imagined. Medicare and Medicaid were introduced to address shortcomings of the private insurance market and now account for a major fraction of total health expenditures. All three programs grew into major programs that resist radical change, and incremental reforms produce effects that are unforeseeable (Weil 2001).

Ultimately, we see no real alternative to a single-payer system or something that approximates it in terms of coordination and rationing. The forces driving health care cost inflation are unlikely to be responsive to increased competition or other market-based approaches (Chernew et al. 2004). Initially, it may be politically necessary to move toward a mixed system such as the one we have today for Medicare, in which the program employs Blue Cross/Blue Shield organizations to review and pay claims. Managed-care organizations, private insurers, and other parties with direct investments in health care financing cannot simply be co-opted or taken over without fair compensation. Initially, we must get past the most serious shortcomings of our current system, especially those that so seriously handicap the working poor and the unemployed. Even as we pursue piecemeal reforms, however, it is important to keep the ultimate objective of a single-payer approach in mind. We suspect that such a system will emerge not from a charitable concern for the uninsured but more from the imperative to introduce economic efficiencies that can help control costs and improve the quality of health care for everyone. Initial state experiments with single-payer programs have produced very positive results that result in significant savings and high-quality care (Shaffer 2003).

Much of the debate surrounding health care financing reform is couched in insurance terminology and the language spoken by health care policy wonks. The term "risk pool" is used to define social categories or groups of people with statistically similar health profiles. Profit-oriented insurers wish to avoid those pools with the greatest need for their services. High-risk individuals and groups become the health insurance wards of the state or do without care. Our families represent a risk pool that is simply unprofitable for private insurers and for whom government programs can be administratively difficult to access. In a single-payer universal health care system, issues of risk would be replaced by considerations of need and the need for medical underwriting eliminated. In effect, we wish to introduce 100 percent "crowd-out," a bit of policy jargon that refers to shifting health care coverage from one program to another or from private plans to the government. What we advocate is moving everyone onto the federal budget.

One major stumbling block in the way of such a universal system and one of the major shortcomings of our present system is its voluntary nature. Americans value their freedom of choice and their right not to participate in programs they do not wish to join or pay into. When it comes to health care, however, voluntary participation is an illusion. We all eventually need care, and a system that allows the young and the healthy to opt out until they are old and sick is neither fair nor economically viable. Health care, like education, is a universal need that everyone is responsible for providing to the community as a collective good. Any equitable and efficient program therefore must be mandatory and, like the tax system, be based on the recognition that just as everyone benefits from public highways, national defense, and the air traffic control system and should help pay for them, everyone benefits from the health care system and should help pay for it.

Health: A Common Good and a Collective Problem

We end this journey by returning to our starting point. Health is clearly a personal asset and something that individuals value highly for themselves and their children. Yet good health is also more than a personal asset and illness more than an individual liability. A healthy population is a national resource upon which everyone's well-being depends. Today's children are tomorrow's workforce, one that will be increasingly African American and Hispanic. Our study state of Texas serves as a prime example of the rapidly changing ethnic face of the labor force and reminds us of the importance of assuring the health of all Americans. Today urban America is becoming increasingly Hispanic (Suro and Singer 2002; U.S. Bureau of the Census 2003b). In the year 2000, 41 percent of Texans between the ages of five and nine were Hispanic, whereas only 17 percent of those over the age of sixty-five were Hispanic (Murdock 2004). These statistics reflect Hispanics' higher fertility and the fact that they are younger on average than non-Hispanics. They also mean that by the year 2040 well over half of the labor force in Texas will be Hispanic. Although the proportion of African Americans and Hispanics differs by state, in most of the rest of the country the working-age population will be disproportionately minority in the relatively short term.

As we noted earlier, if Social Security remains a pay-as-you-go system, the workers of the future will have to contribute an ever-larger fraction of their earnings to support a growing older population (Bongaarts 2004). They will also have to pay for defense, scientific research, the space program, the upgrading of our decaying urban infrastructure, education for the young, medical care, and the rest of the necessities of an advanced developed society. Even if the financing of Social Security were to be changed to rely more on personal investment accounts, the economy is by its very nature a pay-as-you-go operation. Except for aging wine and the petroleum reserve, almost everything that is produced is consumed almost immediately. Savings, investments, and the rest of what constitutes national wealth mean little without workers who have high levels of human capital and are capable of making full use of physical capital. High-skill and demanding jobs require healthy and educated workers. As globalization and international economic competition increase, our national prosperity depends on an ever more productive labor force. If a large segment of that labor force consists of minority Americans who are restricted to low-wage occupations because of health and education disadvantages in youth, the productivity we desperately need will not be there when we need it most.

As our study demonstrates, the major risks to health and barriers to continuous high-quality preventive and acute care are not equally shared by all segments of the population. Minority Americans are more likely than non-Hispanic whites to find themselves living in poverty and to suffer its negative health consequences, and those at the bottom of the economic hierarchy receive lower-quality care than middle-class Americans. Such a situation places the nation in serious jeopardy, and we must at least begin the process of fully incorporating the disadvantaged into the economic mainstream. To that end, adequate lifelong health care is essential.

The basic nature of the health care system we envision can be seen in current experiments with managed care. Today, over half of Medicaid recipients are enrolled in a range of managed-care arrangements (Kaiser Commission 2001). Medicare has also experimented with managed care, with somewhat less success. Nonetheless, the basics of managed care, which include capitation or a predetermined payment for each member of an insured group, and the potential cost-containment devices that such arrangements use are clearly necessary. The potential for coordination and cost control that was part of the initial impetus for managed care is still there. In addition, the basic philosophy of health maintenance and comprehensive care is compatible with universality and full inclusion. In the future, policy debates and experiments with health care delivery will focus on the basic package of care that could be offered all citizens and what fraction of the cost will be paid through taxes and by individual contributions.

Ideally, prevention should be less costly than cure, especially for the chronic conditions that accompany aging, the onset of which can be postponed with appropriate preventive care. Fortunately, the most basic preventive care for pregnant women, infants, children, and even adults is relatively inexpensive. Complex procedures for dealing with cardiovascular disease or cancer are not, and as the population ages and the number of expensive medical innovations increases, the rationing of such care will no doubt become necessary. Many of the most costly problems occur late in life, and their treatment adds significantly to medical care inflation. In the future, we will have no choice but to debate the question of when and how much medical care should be expended on people whose quality of life may not be greatly improved. The rationing of health care may strike some as barbarous, but it occurs daily. Today it is based on the ability to pay, and the poor and minorities find that they are given a smaller share than the more affluent and majority Americans. Tomorrow the inevitable rationing of a scarce and valuable resource will, we hope, be based on a more complex and more equitable set of considerations. Again, our concern is that the poor and minorities not be the first to be denied the care they need.

References

Aaron, Henry J. 1991. *Serious and Unstable Condition: Financing America's Health Care*. Washington, DC: The Brookings Institution.

Acs, Gregory, Pamela Loprest, and Tracy Roberts. 2001. "Final Synthesis Report of Findings from the ASPE 'Leavers' Grants." Report Submitted to the Office of the Assistant Secretary for Planning and Evaluation, U.S. Department of Health and Human Services. Washington, DC: The Urban Institute.

Aday, Lu Ann, G. V. Fleming, and Ronald Andersen. 1984. *Access to Medical Care in the U.S.: Who Has It, Who Doesn't*. Chicago: Pluribus Press.

Adler, Nancy, and Katherine Newman. 2002. "Socioeconomic Disparities in Health: Pathways and Policies." *Health Affairs* 21: 60–77.

Albert, Vicky, and Sandra Catlin. 2002. "Strategic Interaction among the States: An In-depth Look at the Welfare 'Race to the Bottom.'" *Social Work Research* 26: 199–216.

Altman, Stuart H., Uwe E. Reinhardt, and Alexandra E. Shields (Eds.). 1998. *The Future U.S. Healthcare System: Who Will Care for the Poor and Uninsured?* Chicago: Health Administration Press.

Anari, Ali, and Mark G. Datzour. 2004. "Monthly Review of the Texas Economy." In *Recon Newsletter*. College Station, TX: Texas A&M University Real Estate Center.

Angel, Ronald J., and Jacqueline L. Angel. 2005. "Diversity and Aging in the United States." In *Handbook of Aging and the Social Sciences*, edited by Robert H. Binstock and Linda K. George, pp. 94–110. New York: Academic Press.

Angel, Ronald J., and Jacqueline L. Angel. 1993. *Painful Inheritance: Health and the New Generation of Fatherless Families*. Madison: University of Wisconsin Press.

1997. *Who Will Care for Us: Aging and Long-Term Care in Multicultural America*. New York: New York University Press.

Angel, Ronald J., Sonia M. Frias, and Terrence D. Hill. 2005. "Determinants of Household Insurance Coverage among Low-Income Families from Boston, Chicago, and San Antonio: Evidence from the Three City Study." *Social Science Quarterly* 86: 1–16.

Angel, Ronald J., and Peggy Thoits. 1987. "The Impact of Culture on the Cognitive Structure of Illness." *Culture, Medicine, and Psychiatry* 11: 23–52.

Angel, Ronald J., and Kristi Williams. 2000. "Cultural Models of Health and Illness." In *Handbook of Multi-cultural Mental Health: Assessment and Treatment of Diverse Populations*, edited by Israel Cuéllar and Freddy A. Paniagua, pp. 25–44. New York: Academic Press.

Angel, Ronald, and Laura Lein. "The Myth of Self-Sufficiency in Health." In *Doing Without: Women and Work after Welfare Reform*, edited by Jane Henrici. Tucson: University of Arizona Press.

Angel, Ronald, Laura Lein, Jane Henrici, and Emily Leventhal. 2001. *Health Insurance for Children and Their Caregivers in Low Income Neighborhoods – Policy Brief 01-2. Welfare, Children, and Families: A Three City Study*. Baltimore: Johns Hopkins University.

Arrow, Kenneth. 1963. "Uncertainty and the Welfare Economics of Medical Care." *American Economic Review* 53: 941–973.

Asher, Robert, and Charles Stephenson (Eds.). 1990. *Labor Divided: Race and Ethnicity in United States Labor Struggles, 1835–1960*. Albany: State University of New York Press.

Autor, David H., Lawrence F. Katz, and Melissa S. Kearney. 2005. "Trends in U.S. Wage Inequality: Re-assessing the Revisionists." Working paper 11627. Cambridge, MA: National Bureau of Economic Research.

Ayanian, John Z., Betsy A. Kohler, Toshi Abe, and Arnold M. Epstein. 1993. "The Relation between Health Insurance Coverage and Clinical Outcomes among Women with Breast Cancer." *The New England Journal of Medicine* 329: 326–331.

Ayanian, John Z., Joel S. Weissman, Eric C. Schneider, Jack A. Ginsburg, and Alan M. Zaslavsky. 2000. "Unmet Health Needs of Uninsured Adults in the United States." *Journal of the American Medical Association* 284: 2061–2069.

Baker, David W., Martin F. Shapiro, and Claudia L. Schur. 2000. "Health Insurance and Access to Care for Symptomatic Conditions." *Archives of Internal Medicine* 160: 1269–1274.

Barker, Kathleen, and Kathleen Christensen (Eds.). 1998. *Contingent Work: American Employment Relations in Transition*. Ithaca, NY: ILR Press of Cornell University Press.

Bastida, Elena, Israel Cuéllar, and Paul Villas. 2001. "Prevalence of Diabetes Mellitus and Related Conditions in a South Texas Mexican American Sample." *Journal of Community Health Nursing* 18: 75–84.

Bauman, Naomi Lopez, and Devon M. Herrick. 2000. *Uninsured in the Lone Star State.* Washington, DC: National Center for Policy Analysis.

Bell, Stephen H. 2001. "Why Are Caseloads Falling?" Discussion Paper No. 01–02 in series Assessing the New Federalism. Washington, DC: The Urban Institute.

Belous, Richard S. 1989. "How Human Resource Systems Adjust to the Shift toward Contingent Workers." *Monthly Labor Review* 112(3): 7–12.

Bergman, David, Claudia Williams, and Cynthia Pernice. 2004. "SCHIP Changes in a Difficult Budget Climate: A Three-State Site Visit Report." Portland, ME: National Academy for State Health Policy.

Berick, Jill Duerr. 1995. *Faces of Poverty: Portraits of Women and Children on Welfare.* New York: Oxford University Press.

Berk, M. L., L. A. Albers, and C. L. Schur. 1996. "The Growth in the U.S. Uninsured Population: Trends in Hispanic Subgroups, 1977 to 1992." *American Journal of Public Health* 86: 572–576.

Bivens, Josh, Robert Scott, and Christian Weller. 2003. "Mending Manufacturing: Reversing Poor Policy Decisions Is the Only Way to End Current Crisis." Briefing Paper. Washington, DC: Economic Policy Institute.

Black, Sandra A., Kyriakos S. Markides, and Laura A. Ray. 2003. "Depression Predicts Increased Incidence of Adverse Health Outcomes in Older Mexican Americans with Type 2 Diabetes." *Diabetes Care* 26: 2822–2828.

Black, Sandra A., Laura A. Ray, and Kyriakos S. Markides. 1999. "The Prevalence and Health Burden of Self-Reported Diabetes in Older Mexican Americans: Findings from the Hispanic Established Populations for Epidemiologic Studies of the Elderly." *American Journal of Public Health* 89: 546–552.

Blackwell, Debra L., Mark D. Hayward, and Eileen. M. Crimmins. 2001. "Does Childhood Health Affect Chronic Morbidity in Later Life?" *Social Science and Medicine* 52: 1269–1284.

Blank, Rebecca M. 2002. "Evaluating Welfare Reform in the United States." *Journal of Economic Literature* 40: 1105–1166.

Blank, Rebecca M., and Lucie Schmidt. 2001. "Work, Wages, and Welfare." In *The New World of Welfare*, edited by Rebecca Blank and Ron Haskins, pp. 70–96. Washington, DC: Brookings Institution Press.

Bluestone, Barry, and Bennett Harrison. 1988. "The Growth of Low-Wage Employment: 1963–86." *The American Economic Review* 78: 124–128.

Blumberg, Linda J., and John Holahan. 2004a. "Changes in Insured Coverage and Access to Care for Middle Class Americans, 1999–2002." *Health Policy On-line*, No. 8. Washington, DC: The Urban Institute. URL:http://www.urban.org./url.cfm?ID – 1000644. Accessed November 9, 2005.

2004b. "Work, Offers, and Take-Up: Decomposing the Source of Recent Declines in Employer-Sponsored Insurance." *Health Policy On-line*, No. 9. Washington, DC: The Urban Institute. URL:http://www.urban.org/url.cfm?ID = 1000645. Accessed November 9, 2005.

Bodenheimer, Thomas. 1990. "Should We Abolish the Private Health Insurance Industry?" *International Journal of Health Services* 20: 199–220.

——— 2003. "The Movement for Universal Health Insurance: Finding Common Ground." *American Journal of Public Health* 93: 112–115.

Bongaarts, John. 2004. "Population Aging and the Rising Cost of Public Pensions." Working Paper No. 185, edited by Policy Research Division. New York: Population Council.

Bonilla-Silva, Eduardo. 2003. *Racism without Racists: Color-Blind Racism and the Persistence of Racial Inequality in the United States*. New York: Rowman and Littlefield.

Bonoli, Giuliano. 2001. "Political Institutions, Veto Points, and the Process of Welfare State Adaptation." In *The New Politics of the Welfare State*, edited by Paul Pierson, pp. 238–264. Oxford: Oxford University Press.

Boslaugh, S., G. Fairbrother, M. Dutton, D. Hyson, and K. Lobach. 1999. "Experiences of Families that Applied for Government-Sponsored Child Health Insurance: Report of a Follow-up Study in New York City." *Journal of Urban Health* 76: 335–350.

Boston Redevelopment Authority. 2001. *Boston's Population–2000: section 6. Population Changes in Boston's Asian and Hispanic Ethnic Groups: 1990–2000*, edited by Boston Redevelopment Authority. Boston: City of Boston.

Boushey, Heather, and David Rosnick. 2004. "Issue Brief: For Welfare Reform to Work, Jobs Must Be Available." Washington, DC: Center for Economic and Policy Research.

Brauner, Sarah, and Pamela J. Loprest. 1999. "Where Are They Now? What States' Studies of People Who Left Welfare Tell Us." In Publication No. A-32 in series New Federalism: Issues and Options for States. Washington, DC: The Urban Institute.

Broaddus, Matthew, and Leighton Ku. 2000. "Nearly 95 Percent of Low-Income Uninsured Children Now Are Eligible for MEDICAID or SCHIP: Measures Need to Increase Enrollment among Eligible but Uninsured Children." Washington, DC: Center on Budget and Policy Priorities.

Browning, Rufus P., Dale Rogers Marshall, and David H. Tabb. 2003. *Racial Politics in American Cities*. New York: Longman.

Bureau of Labor Statistics. 2004a. "BLS Releases 2002–12 Employment Projections." USDL 04–148. Washington, DC: U.S. Department of Labor. URL: http:// stats.bls.gov.news.release/ecopro.nro.htm. Accessed November 9, 2005.

——— 2004b. "Manufacturing." NAICS 31–33. In *Industry at a Glance*. Washington, DC: U.S. Department of Labor. URL: http://www.bls.gov/iag/manufacturing.htm. Accessed November 9, 2005.

Burton, Linda, Andrew J. Cherlin, Judith Francis, Robin Jarrett, James Quane, Constance Williams, and N. Michelle Stem Cook. 1998. "What Welfare Recipients and the Fathers of Their Children Are Saying about Welfare

Reform, June 1998." In *Welfare, Children & Families: A Three City Study*, Baltimore: Johns Hopkins University.

Burton, Linda M., Laura Lein, and Amy Kolak. 2005. "'The Walls of Jericho': Health and Mothers' Employment in Low-Income Families." In *Work, Family, Health, and Well-Being*, edited by Suzanne M. Bianchi, Lynne M. Casper, and Rosalind Berkowitz King, pp. 493–510. Mahwah, NJ: Lawrence Erlbaum.

Burton, Linda M., and Keith E. Whitfield. 2003. "'Weathering' Toward Poorer Health in Later Life: Co-morbidity in Low-Income Urban Families." *Public Policy and Aging Report* 13: 13–18.

Burton, Linda M., Robin Jarrett, Laura Lein, Steven Matthews, James Quane, Deborah Skinner, Constance Williams, William J. Wilson, and T. Hurt. 2001. *"Structured Discovery": Ethnography, Welfare Reform and the Assessment of Neighborhoods, Families and Children*. Minneapolis, MN: Society for Research on Child Development.

Butler, Patricia. 2000a. *ERISA Preemption Primer*. Washington, DC: Academy Health.

Butler, Patricia A. 2000b. "ERISA and State Health Care Access Initiatives: Opportunites and Obstacles." New York: The Commonwealth Fund.

Capps, Randolph, Michael E. Fix, and Jeffrey S. Passel. 2003. "A Profile of the Low-Wage Immigrant Workforce." In Brief No. 4 in series Immigrant Families and Workers: Facts and Perspectives. Washington, DC: The Urban Institute.

Capps, Randolph, Nancy M. Pindus, Kathleen Snyder, and Jacob Leos-Urbel. 2001. "Recent Changes in Texas Welfare and Work, Child Care and Child Welfare Systems, State Update No. 1." In series Assessing the New Federalism. Washington, DC: The Urban Institute.

Capps, Randy. 2001. "Hardship among Children of Immigrants: Findings from the 1999 National Survey of American Families." Publication No. B-29 in series New Federalism: National Survey of America's Families. Washington, DC: The Urban Institute.

Carrasquillo, Olveen, Angeles Carrasquillo, and Steven Shea. 2000. "Health Insurance Coverage Immigrants Living in the United States: Differences by Citizenship Status and Country of Origin." *American Journal of Public Health* 90: 917–923.

Carter, Jannette S., Jacqueline A. Pugh, and Ana Monterrosa. 1996. "Non-Insulin-Dependent Diabetes Mellitus in Minorities in the United States." *Annals of Internal Medicine* 125: 221–232.

Centers for Disease Control. 1999. "Ten Great Public Health Achievements – United States, 1900–1999." *Morbidity and Mortality Weekly Report* 48: 241–243.

Chavkin, Wendy, Diana Romero, and Paul Wise. 2000. "State Welfare Reform Policies and Declines in Health Insurance." *American Journal of Public Health* 90: 900–908.

Chavkin, Wendy, and Paul Wise. 2002. "The Data Are In: Health Matters in Welfare Policy." *American Journal of Public Health* 92: 1392–1396.

Chernew, Michael E., Peter D. Jacobson, Timothy P. Hofer, Keith D. Aaronson, and A. Mark Fendrick. 2004. "Barriers to Constraining Health Care Cost Growth." *Health Affairs* 23: 122–128.

Child Trends Data Bank. 2003. "Health Care Coverage." Available at: http://www.childtrendsdatabank.org/indicators/26HealthCareCoverage. cfm. Accessed November 9, 2005.

Chollet, Deborah. 1994. "Employer-Based Health Insurance in a Changing Work Force." *Health Affairs* 13: 315–326.

Chu, Susan Y., Lawrence E. Barker, and Philip J. Smith. 2004. "Racial/Ethnic Disparities in Preschool Immunizations: United States, 1996–2001." *American Journal of Public Health* 94: 973–977.

Claxton, Gary, Isadora Gil, Ben Finder, Erin Holve, Jon Gabel, Jeremy Pickreign, Heidi Whitmore, Samantha Hawkins, and Cheryl Fahlman. 2004. "Employer Health Benefits, 2004 Annual Survey." In *Health Care Marketplace Project*. Menlo Park, CA: Henry J. Kaiser Family Foundation and Health Research and Educational Trust.

Collins, Sara R., Cathy Schoen, Diane Colasanto, and Derdre A. Downey. 2003. *On the Edge: Low-Wage Workers and Their Health Insurance Coverage: Findings from the Commonwealth Fund 2001 Health Insurance Survey*. Washington, DC: The Commonwealth Fund.

Committee on Assuring the Health of the Public in the 21st Century. 2002. *The Future of the Public's Health in the 21st Century*. Washington, DC: National Academy of Sciences.

Committee on Child Health Financing. 2001. "Implementation Principles and Strategies for the State Children's Health Insurance Program." *Pediatrics* 107: 1214–1220.

Congressional Budget Office. 2004. "What Accounts for the Decline in Manufacturing Employment?" Economic and Budget Issue Brief. Washington, DC: Congressional Budget Office.

Cooper, Philip F., and Barbara S. Schone. 1997. "More Offers, Fewer Takers for Employment-Based Health Insurance: 1987 and 1996." *Health Affairs* 16: 142–149.

Cornelius, L. J. 1993. "Ethnic Minorities and Access to Medical Care: Where Do They Stand?" *Journal of the Association for Academic Minority Physicians* 4: 16–25.

Cunningham, Peter J. 2003. "SCHIP Making Progress: Increased Take-up Contributes to Coverage Gains." *Health Affairs* 22: 163–172.

———. 2005. "Medicaid Cost Containment and Access to Prescription Drugs: States' Efforts to Contain the Rising Costs of Medicaid Prescription Drugs Are Reducing Enrollees' Access to Needed Medications." *Health Affairs* 24: 780–789.

Cunningham, Peter J., and Michael H. Park. 2001. "Recent Trends in Children's Health Insurance: No Gains for Low-Income Children." Issue Brief No. 29. Washington, DC: Center for Studying Health System Change.

Cunningham, Robert III, and Robert M. Cunningham, Jr. 1997. *The Blues: A History of the Blue Cross and Blue Shield System*. De Kalb: Northern Illinois University Press.

Curtis, Richard E., Edward Neuschler, and Rafe Forland. 2001. "Consumer-Choice Purchasing Pools: Past Tense, Future Perfect? These Pools Could Play an Important Role in Securing Coverage for American Workers." *Health Affairs* 20: 164–168.

Daniels, Norman, Donald W. Light, and Ronald C. Caplan. 1996. *Benchmarks of Fairness for Health Care Reform*. Oxford: Oxford University Press.

Danziger, Sandra, Mary Corcoran, Sheldon Danziger, Colleen Heflin, Ariel Kalil, Judy Levine, Daniel Rosen, Kristin Seefeldt, Kristine Siefert, and Richard Tolman. 2000. *Barriers to Employment of Welfare Recipients*. Ann Arbor: University of Michigan Poverty Research and Training Center.

Danziger, Sheldon H., and Robert H. Haveman (Eds.). 2001. *Understanding Poverty*. New York and Cambridge, MA: Russell Sage Foundation and Harvard University Press.

Davidoff, Amy, A. Garrett, Diane Makuc, and Mathew Schirmer. 2000. "Medicaid-Eligible Children Who Don't Enroll: Health Status, Access to Care, and Implications for Medicaid Enrollment." *Inquiry* 37: 203–218.

Davidoff, Amy J., Bowen Garrett, and Matthew Schirmer. 2000. "Children Eligible for Medicaid but Not Enrolled: How Great a Policy Concern?" Publication No. A-41 in series New Federalism: Issues and Options for States. Washington, DC: Urban Institute.

Davidoff, Amy, Anna S. Sommers, Jennifer Lesko, and Alshadye Yemane. 2004. *Medicaid and State-Funded Coverage for Adults: Estimates of Eligibility and Enrollment*. Report No. 7078. The Kaiser Commission on Medicaid and the Uninsured. Washington, DC: The Henry J. Kaiser Family Foundation.

Davies, Gareth, and Martha Derthick. 1997. "Race and Social Welfare Policy: The Social Security Act of 1935." *Political Science Quarterly* 112: 217–235.

Davis, Karen, and Cathy Schoen. 2003. "Creating Consensus on Coverage Choices." *Health Affairs*, 10. 1377/hlthaff.w3.199.

Davis, Karen, Cathy Schoen, and Stephen C. Schoenbaum. 2000. "A 2020 Vision for American Health Care." *Archives of Internal Medicine* 160: 3357–3362.

De la Torre, Adela, Robert Friis, Harold R. Hunter, and Lorena Garcia. 1996. "The Health Insurance Status of U.S. Latino Women: A Profile from the 1982–84 HHANES." *American Journal of Public Health* 86: 533–537.

DeNavas-Walt, Carmen, Bernadette D. Proctor, and Robert J. Mills. 2004. "Income, Poverty, and Health Insurance Coverage in the United States: 2003." In *U.S. Census Bureau, Current Population Reports, Series P60–226*. Washington, DC: U.S. Government Printing Office.

Didrickson, Loleta A. 1997. "Illinois Employment Trends – Largest Increase in Jobs in Service Sector." *Fiscal Focus*, pp. 1 and 6–7, March 1997. Office of Illinois Comptroller, Springfield : State of Illinois.

Diehl, A. K., and M. K. Stern. 1989. "Special Health Problems of Mexican-Americans: Obesity, Gallbladder Disease, Diabetes Mellitus, and Cardiovascular Disease." *Advances in Internal Medicine* 34: 73–96.

Dohrenwend, B. P., P. E. Shrout, G. Egri, and F. S. Mendelsohn. 1980. "Nonspecific Psychological Distress and Other Dimensions of Psychopathology. Measures for Use in the General Population." *Archives of General Psychiatry* 37: 1229–1236.

Doty, Michelle M. 2003. "Hispanic Patients' Double Burden: Lack of Health Insurance and Limited English." Publication Number 592. New York: The Commonwealth Fund.

Doty, M. M., and B. L. Ives. 2002. "Quality of Health Care for Hispanic Populations: Findings from The Commonwealth Fund 2001." *Health Care Quality Survey*, Publication Number 526. New York: The Commonwealth Fund.

Dubay, Lisa, Jennifer M. Haley, and Genevieve M. Kenney. 2002. "Children's Eligibility for Medicaid and SCHIP: A View from 2000." Publication No. B-41 in series New Federalism: National Survey of America's Families. Washington, DC: The Urban Institute.

Dunkelberg, Anne, and Molly O'Malley. 2004. *Children's Medicaid and SCHIP in Texas: The Impact of Budget Cuts*. Report No. 7123. The Kaiser Commission on Medicaid and the Uninsured. Washington, DC: The Henry J. Kaiser Family Foundation.

Edin, Kathryn, and Maria Kefalas. 2005. *Promises I Can Keep: Why Poor Women Put Motherhood Before Marriage*. Berkeley: University of California Press.

Edin, Kathryn, and Laura Lein. 1997. *Making Ends Meet: How Single Mothers Survive Welfare and Low-Wage Work*. New York: Russell Sage Foundation.

Elixhauser, A., S. Machlin, M. Zodet, F. Chevarley, N. Patel, M. McCormick, and L. Simpson. 2002. "Health Care for Children and Youth in the United States: 2001 Annual Report on Access, Utilization, Quality, and Expenditures." *Ambulatory Pediatrics* 2: 419–437.

Elwood, D., R. Blank, J. Blasi, D. Krase, W. Niskanen, and K. Lynne-Dyson. 2000. *A Working Nation: Workers, Work and Government in the New Economy*. New York: Russell Sage Foundation.

Enthoven, Alain C. 1979. "Consumer-Centered vs. Job-Centered Health Insurance." *Harvard Business Review* 57: 141–152.

Esping-Andersen, Gøsta. 1990. *The Three Worlds of Welfare Capitalism.* Princeton, NJ: Princeton University Press.

——— 1999. *Social Foundations of Postindustrial Economies.* Oxford: Oxford University Press.

Esping-Andersen, Gøsta, Duncan Gallie, Anton Hemerijck, and John Myles. 2002. *Why We Need a New Welfare State.* Oxford: Oxford University Press.

Farber, H. S., and H. Levy. 2000. "Recent Trends in Employer-Sponsored Health Insurance Coverage: Are Bad Jobs Getting Worse?" *Journal of Health Economics* 19: 93–119.

Feder, Judith, Larry Levitt. 2001. "Covering the Low-Income Uninsured: The Case for Expanding Public Programs." *Health Affairs* 20: 27–39.

Fein, Rashi. 1986. *Medical Care, Medical Costs.* Cambridge, MA: Harvard University Press.

Finch, Brian Karl, Bohdan Kolody, and William A. Vega. 2000. "Perceived Discrimination and Depression among Mexican-Origin Adults in California." *Journal of Health and Social Behavior* 41: 295–313.

Flora, Peter (Ed.). 1986. *Growth to Limits: The European Social Welfare States since World War II.* Berlin: Walter de Gruyter.

Flores, Glenn, M. Abreu, M. A. Olivar, and B. Kastner. 1998. "Access Barriers to Health Care for Latino Children." *Archives of Pediatrics and Adolescent Medicine* 152: 1119–1125.

Flores, Glenn, Elena Fuentes-Afflick, Oxiris Barbot, Olivia Carter-Pokras, Luz Claudio, Marielena Lara, Jennie A. McLaurin, Lee Pachter, Francisco Ramos Gomez, Fernando Mendoza, R. Burciaga Valdez, Antonia M. Villarruel, Ruth E. Zambrana, Robert Greenberg, and Michael Weitzman. 2002. "The Health of Latino Children: Urgent Priorities, Unanswered Questions, and a Research Agenda." *Journal of the American Medical Association* 288: 82–90.

Fox, Daniel M. 1986. *Health Policies, Health Politics: British and American Experience, 1911–1965.* Princeton, NJ: Princeton University Press.

Freeman, Howard E., Linda H. Aiken, Robert J. Blendon, and Christopher R. Corey. 1990. "Uninsured Working-Age Adults: Characteristics and Consequences." *Health Services Research* 24: 811–823.

Freeman, Richard B. 2001. "The Rising Tide Lifts?" In *Understanding Poverty*, edited by Sheldon H. Danziger and Robert H. Haveman, pp. 97–126. New York and Cambridge, MA: Russell Sage Foundation and Harvard University Press.

Freund, Peter E. S., Meredith B. McGuire, and Linda S. Podhurst. 2003. *Health, Illness, and the Social Body: A Critical Sociology.* Upper Saddle River, NJ: Prentice-Hall.

Gabel, Jon, Gary Claxton, Erin Holve, Jeremy Pickreign, Heidi Whitmore, Kelley Dhont, Samantha Hawkins, and Diane Rowland. 2003. "Health Benefits in 2003: Premiums Reach Thirteen-Year High as

Employers Adopt New Forms of Cost Sharing." *Health Affairs* 22: 117–126.

Garey, Anita Ilta. 1999. *Weaving Work and Motherhood*. Philadelphia: Temple University Press.

Geronimus, Arlene T. 1996. "Black/White Differences in the Relationship of Maternal Age to Birthweight: A Population-Based Test of the Weathering Hypothesis." *Social Science and Medicine* 42: 589–597.

Giachello, A. L. 1992. "Hispanics and Health Care." In *Hispanics in the United States*, edited by P. S. Cafferty and W. C. McCready, pp. 159–194. New Brunswick, NJ: Transaction Publishers.

Gilbert, Neil, and Barbara Gilbert. 1989. *The Enabling State: Modern Welfare Capitalism in America*. Oxford: Oxford University Press.

Gilens, Martin. 1999. *Why Americans Hate Welfare: Race, Media and the Politics of Antipoverty Policy*. Chicago: University of Chicago Press.

Gilmer, Todd, and Richard Kronick. 2005. "It's the Premiums, Stupid: Projections of the Uninsured through 2013." *Health Affairs,* 10.1377/hlthaff.w5.143.

Glaeser, Edward L., Eric A. Hanuskek, and John M. Quigley. 2004. "Opportunities, Race, and Urban Location: The Influence of John Kain." *Journal of Urban Economics* 56: 70–79.

Golden, Miriam A., Michael Wallerstein, and Peter Lange. 1999. "Postwar Trade-Union Organization and Industrial Relations in Twelve Countries." In *Continuity and Change in Contemporary Capitalism*, edited by Herbert Kitschelt, Peter Lange, Gary Marks, and John D. Stephens, pp. 194–230. Cambridge: Cambridge University Press.

Goldscheider, Francis K., and Calvin Goldscheider. 1991. "The Intergenerational Flow of Income: Family Structure and the Status of Black Americans." *Journal of Marriage and the Family* 53: 499–508.

Goodman, John C. 2001. "Characteristics of an Ideal Health Care System." NCP A Policy Report No. 242. Washington, DC: Center for Policy Analysis.

Goodwin, Doris Kearns. 1991. *Lyndon Johnson and the American Dream*. New York: St. Martin's Press.

Goodwin, Joanne L. 1997. *Gender and the Politics of Welfare Reform: Mothers' Pensions in Chicago, 1911–1929*. Chicago: University of Chicago Press.

Gottschalk, Marie. 2000. *The Shadow Welfare State: Labor, Business, and the Politics of Health-Care in the United States*. Ithaca, NY: ILR Press.

Gottschalk, Peter, and Timothy M. Smeeding. 2000. "Empirical Evidence on Income Inequality in Industrialized Countries." In *Handbook of Income Distribution*, edited by Anthony B. Atkinson and François Bourguignon, pp. 261–308. New York: Elsevier-North-Holland.

Granados, Gilberto, Puwula Jyoti, Nancy Berman, and Patrick T. Dowling. 2001. "Health Care for Latino Children: Impact of Child and Parental Birthplace on Insurance Status and Access to Health Services." *American Journal of Public Health* 91: 1806–1807.

Grebler, Leo, Joan W. Moore, and Ralph C. Guzman. 1970. *The Mexican-American People: The Nation's Second Largest Minority*. New York: The Free Press.

Grogger, Jeffrey, and Stephen J. Trejo. 2002. *Falling Behind or Moving Up? The Intergenerational Progress of Mexican Americans*. San Francisco: Public Policy Institute of California.

Guzmán, Betsy. 2001. "The Hispanic Population 2000." Report No. C2KBR/01–3. *Census 2000 Brief*. Washington, DC: U.S. Bureau of the Census.

Gutkovich, Zinoviy, Richard N. Rosenthal, Igor Galynker, Christopher Muran, Sarai Batchelder, and Elena Itskhoki. 1999. "Depression and Demoralization among Russian-Jewish Immigrants in Primary Care." *Psychosomatics* 40: 117–125.

Guyer, Jocelyn. 2000. "Health Care after Welfare: An Update of Findings from State-Level Leaver Studies." Washington, DC: Center for Budget and Policy Priorities.

Hacker, Jacob S. 1997. *The Road to Nowhere: The Genesis of President Clinton's Plan for Health Security*. Princeton, NJ: Princeton University Press.

——— 2002. *The Divided Welfare State*. New York: Cambridge University Press.

Hadley, Jack. 2004. "Labor Force Status and Insurance Coverage, 1999 and 2002." In *Health Policy On-line*, No. 7. Washington, DC: The Urban Institute. URL: http://www.urban.org/url.cfm?ID=1000643. Accessed November 10, 2005.

Haley, Jennifer M., and Stephen Zuckerman. 2000. "Health Insurance, Access, and Use: United States. Tabulations from the 1997 National Survey of America's Families." In *Assessing the New Federalism*. Washington, DC: The Urban Institute. URL: http://www.urban.org/UploadedPDF/discussion 00-14.pdf. Accessed November 10, 2005.

Halfon, N. D., L. Wood, R. B. Valdez, M. Pereyra, and N. Duan. 1997. "Medicaid Enrollment and Health Services Access by Latino Children in Inner City Los Angeles." *Journal of the American Medical Association* 277: 636–641.

Hanson, Karla. 2001. "Patterns of Insurance Coverage within Families with Children." *Health Affairs* 20: 240–246.

Harris, M. I., K. M. Flegal, C. C. Cowie, M. S. Eberhardt, D. E. Goldstein, R. R. Little, H. M. Wiedmeyer, and D. D. Byrd-Holt. 1998. "Prevalence of Diabetes, Impaired Fasting Glucose, and Impaired Glucose Tolerance in U.S. Adults. The Third National Health and Nutrition Examination Survey, 1988–1994." *Diabetes Care* 21: 518–524.

Hays, Sharon. 2003. *Flat Broke with Children: Women in the Age of Welfare Reform.* New York: Oxford University Press.

Health Care Financing Administration. 2000. *A Profile of Medicaid: Chartbook 2000.* Washington, DC: U.S. Department of Health and Human Services.

Heck, Katherine E., and Jennifer D. Parker. 2002. "Family Structure, Socioeconomic Status and Access to Health Care for Children." *Health Services Research* 37: 173–186.

Heclo, Hugh. 1995. "The Social Question." In *Poverty, Inequality, and the Future of Social Policy: Western States in the New World Order*, edited by Katherine McFate, Roger Lawson, and William Julius Wilson, pp. 665–691. New York: Russell Sage Foundation.

——— 2001. "The Politics of Welfare Reform." In *The New World of Welfare*, edited by Rebecca M. Blank and Ron Haskins, pp. 169–200. Washington, DC: Brookings Institution Press.

Hedley, Allison A., Cynthia L. Ogden, Clifford L. Johnson, Margaret D. Carroll, Lester R. Curtin, and Katherine M. Flegal. 2004. "Prevalence of Overweight and Obesity among US Children, Adolescents, and Adults, 1999–2002." *Journal of the American Medical Association* 291: 2847–2850.

Henly, Julia R., and Sandra Lyons. 2000. "The Negotiations of Child Care and Employment Demands among Low-Income Parents." *Journal of Social Issues* 56: 683–705.

Heymann, Jody. 2000. *The Widening Gap: Why America's Working Families Are in Jeopardy and What Can Be Done About It.* New York: Basic Books.

Hicks, Alexander. 1999. *Social Democracy and Welfare Capitalism.* Ithaca, NY: Cornell University Press.

Hill, Ian, and Amy Westpfahl Lutzky. 2003. "Getting in, Not Getting in, and Why: Understanding SCHIP Enrollment." Assessing the New Federalism Occasional Paper No. 66. Washington, DC: The Urban Institute.

Himmelstein, David U., Elizabeth Warren, Deborah Thorne, and Steffie Woolhandler. 2005. "MarketWatch: Illness and Injury as Contributors to Bankruptcy." *Health Affairs Web Exclusive*; 10.1377/hlthaff.w5.63, February 2, 2005.

Himmelstein, David U., and Steffie Woolhandler. 2003. "National Health Insurance or Incremental Reform: Aim High, or at Our Feet?" *American Journal of Public Health* 93: 102–105.

Hoadley, John F., Peter J. Cunningham, and Megan McHugh. 2004. "Popular Medicaid Programs Do Battle with State Budget Pressures: Perspectives from Twelve States." *Health Affairs* 23: 143–154.

Hoelscher, Deanna M., R. Sue Day, Eun Sul Lee, Ralph F. Frankowski, Steven H. Kelder, Jerri L. Ward, and Michael E. Scheurer. 2004. "Measuring the Prevalence of Overweight in Texas Schoolchildren." *American Journal of Public Health* 94: 1002–1008.

Hoffman, Beatrix Rebecca. 2001. *The Wages of Sickness: The Politics of Health Insurance in Progressive America*. Chapel Hill: University of North Carolina Press.

Holahan, John, and Brian Bruen. 2003. "Medicaid Spending: What Factors Contributed to the Growth between 2000 and 2002?" Washington, DC: The Urban Institute.

Holl, Jane L., Kristen Shook Slack, and Amy Bush Stevens. 2005. "Welfare Reform and Health Insurance: Consequences for Parents." *American Journal of Public Health* 95: 279–285.

Howard, Christopher. 1997. *The Hidden Welfare State: Tax Expenditures and Social Policy in the United States*. Princeton, NJ: Princeton University Press.

Hubble, F., H. Waitzkin, S. Mishra, and L. Chavez. 1991. "Access to Medical Care for Documented and Undocumented Latinos in a Southern California County." *Western Journal of Medicine* 154: 414–417.

Huber, Evelyne, and John D. Stephens. 2001a. *Development and Crisis of the Welfare State: Parties and Policies in Global Markets*. Chicago: University of Chicago Press.

2001b. "Welfare State and Production Regimes in the Era of Retrenchment." In *The New Politics of the Welfare State*, edited by Paul Pierson, pp. 107–145. Oxford: Oxford University Press.

Iannotta, J. G. (Ed.). 2002. *Emerging Issues in Hispanic Health: Summary of a Workshop*. Washington, DC: National Academy Press.

Institute of Medicine. 2001. *Coverage Matters: Insurance and Health Care*. Washington, DC: National Academy Press.

2002a. *Care without Coverage: Too Little, Too Late*. Washington, DC: National Academy Press.

2002b. *Health Insurance Is a Family Matter*. Washington, DC: National Academy Press.

2003a. *Hidden Costs, Value Lost: Uninsurance in America*. Washington, DC: National Academy Press.

2003b. *A Shared Destiny: Community Effects of Uninsurance*. Washington, DC: National Academy Press.

2004. *Insuring America's Health: Principles and Recommendations*. Washington, DC: National Academy Press.

Isaacs, Julia B., and Matthew R. Lyon. 2000. "A Cross-State Examination of Families Leaving Welfare: Findings from the ASPE-Funded Leavers Studies." Paper presented at the National Association for Welfare Research and Statistics (NAWRS) 40th Annual Workshop, Scottsdale, AZ. Washington, DC: Office of the Assistant Secretary for Planning and Evaluation, U.S. Department of Health and Human Services.

Jackson, James S., Tony N. Brown, David R. Williams, Myriam Torres, Sherrill L. Sellers, and Kendrick Brown. 1996. "Racism and the Physical and Mental Health Status of African Americans: A Thirteen Year National Panel Study." *Ethnicity and Disease* 6: 132–147.

Jacoby, Melissa, Teresa A. Sullivan, and Elizabeth Warren. 2000. "Medi-
cal Problems and Bankruptcy Filings." *Norton Bankruptcy Law Adviser*
May: 1–12.
　2001. "Rethinking the Debates over Health Care Financing: Evidence
from the Bankruptcy Courts." *New York University Law Review* 76:
375–418.
Jayakody, Rukmalie, Sheldon Danziger, and Harold Pollack. 2000. "Welfare
Reform, Substance Use, and Mental Health." *Journal of Health, Politics,
Policy, and Law* 24: 623–651.
Kahn, Charles N., III, and Ronald F. Pollack. 2001. "Building a Consensus for
Expanding Health Coverage." *Health Affairs* 20: 40–48.
Kain, John F., and John M. Quigley. 1972. "Housing Market Discrimination,
Homeownership, and Savings Behavior." *American Economic Review* 62:
263–277.
Kaiser Commission. 2001. "Medicaid and Managed Care." Fact Sheet:2068-
3. The Kaiser Commission on Medicaid and the Uninsured. Washington,
DC: The Henry J. Kaiser Family Foundation.
Kaiser Commission. 2004. *Trends and Indicators in the Changing Health Care
Marketplace, 2004 Update: Information Provided by the Health Care
Marketplace Project Publication No. 7031.* Washington, DC: The Henry
J. Kaiser Family Foundation.
Kaiser Commission on Medicaid and the Uninsured. 2003. *The Health Insur-
ance Status of Low-Income Children and Their Parents: Recent Trends in
Coverage and State-Level Data.* Washington, DC: Henry J. Kaiser Family
Foundation.
Kalleberg, A., B. Reskin, and K. Hudson. 2000. "Bad Jobs in America: Stan-
dard and Nonstandard Employment Relations and Job Quality in the
United States." *American Sociological Review* 65: 256–278.
Kasper, Judith, Terence Giovannini, and Catherine Hoffman. 2000. "Gain-
ing and Losing Health Insurance: Strengthening the Evidence for Effects
on Access to Care and Health Outcomes." *Medical Care Research and
Review* 57: 298–318.
Katz, Michael B. 2001. *The Price of Citizenship: Redefining the American
Welfare State.* New York: Henry Holt and Company.
Kazis, Richard, and Marc S. Miller (Eds.). 2001. *Low-Wage Workers in the
New Economy.* Washington, DC: The Urban Institute.
Kenney, Genevieve M., Jennifer M. Haley, and Alexandra Tebay. 2003.
"Children's Insurance Coverage and Service Use Improve." Washington,
DC: The Urban Institute.
Kessler, Ronald C., Kristin D. Mickelson, and David R. Williams. 1999. "The
Prevalence, Distribution, and Mental Health Correlates of Perceived Dis-
crimination in the United States." *Journal of Health and Social Behavior*
40: 208–230.

King, Desmond, and Stewart Wood. 1999. "The Political Economy of Neoliberalism: Britain and the United States in the 1980s." In *Continuity and Change in Contemporary Capitalism*, edited by Herbert Kitschelt, Peter Lange, Gary Marks, and John D. Stephens, pp. 371–397. Cambridge: Cambridge University Press.

Kingfisher, Catherine Pelissier. 1996. *Women in the American Welfare Trap*. Philadelphia: University of Pennsylvania Press.

Kingston, Richard S. 2002. "Why Exploiting This Knowledge Will Be Essential to Achieving Health Improvements in the 21st Century." In *Through the Kaleidoscope: Viewing the Contributions of the Behavioral and Social Sciences to Health*, edited by Lisa F. Berkman, pp. 24–28. Washington, DC: National Academy Press.

Kitschelt, Herbert, Peter Lange, Gary Marks, and John D. Stephens (Eds.). 1999. *Continuity and Change in Contemporary Capitalism*. Cambridge: Cambridge University Press.

Koivusalo, Meri Tuulikki. 2005. "The Future of European Health Policies." *International Journal of Health Services* 35: 325–342.

Kreiger, Nancy, Stephen Sidney, and Eugenie Coakley. 1999. "Racial Discrimination and Skin Color in the CARDIA Study: Implications for Public Health Research." *American Journal of Public Health* 88: 1308–1313.

Ku, Leighton, and Shannon Blaney. 2000. "Health Coverage for Legal Immigrant Children: New Census Data Highlight Importance of Restoring Medicaid and SCHIP Coverage." Washington, DC: Center for Budget and Policy Priorities.

Ku, Leighton, and Brian Bruen. 2000. "The Continuing Decline in Medicaid Coverage." Publication No. A-37 in series The New Federalism: Issues and Options for States. Washington, DC: The Urban Institute.

Ku, Leighton, and Timothy Waidmann. 2003. *How Race/Ethnicity, Immigration Status and Language Affect Health Insurance Coverage, Access to Care and Quality of Care among the Low-Income Population*. Publication No. 4132. The Kaiser Commission on Medicaid and the Uninsured. New York: The Henry J. Kaiser Family Foundation.

Kuo, Yong-Fang, Mukaila A. Raji, Kyriakos S. Markides, Laura A. Ray, David V. Espino, and James A. Goodwin. 2003. "Inconsistent Use of Diabetes Medications, Diabetes Complications, and Mortality in Older Mexican Americans over a 7-Year Period: Data from the Hispanic Established Population for the Epidemiologic Study of the Elderly." *Diabetes Care* 26: 3054–3060.

Lambert, Susan, E. Waxman, and A. Haley-Lock. 2002. "Against the Odds: A Study Sources of Instability in Lower-Skilled Jobs." Working Paper of the Project on the Public Economy of Work. Chicago: Univeristy of Chicago, School of Social Service Administration.

Lee, Geum-Yong, and Ronald J. Angel. 2002. "Living Arrangements and Supplemental Security Income Use among Elderly Asians and Hispanics in the United States: The Role of Nativity and Citizenship." *Journal of Ethnic and Migration Studies* 28: 553–563.

Lee, Ronald. 1997. "Public Costs of Long Life and Low Fertility: Will the Baby Boomers Break the Budget?" Berkeley: Resource Center on Aging, University of California.

Lein, Laura, Alan F. Benjamin, Monica McManus, and Kevin Roy. 2005. " 'Economic Roulette': When Is a Job Not a Job?" *Community, Work and Family* 8: 359–378.

Lesser, Cara S., and Paul B. Ginsburg. 2003. "Health Care Cost and Access Problems Intensify: Initial Findings from HSC's Recent Site Visits." Issue Brief No. 63. Washington, DC: Center for Studying Health System Change.

Lewis, Oscar. 1959. *Five Families; Mexican Case Studies in the Culture of Poverty*. New York: New American Library.

    1966. *La Vida: A Puerto Rican Family in the Culture of Poverty – San Juan and New York*. New York: Random House.

Lieberman, Robert C. 1998. *Shifting the Color Line: Race and the American Welfare State*. Cambridge, MA: Harvard University Press.

Light, Donald W. 1992. "The Practice and Ethics of Risk-Rated Health Insurance." *Journal of the American Medical Association* 267: 2503–2508.

Lillie-Blanton, Marsha D., Wilhelmina A. Leigh, and Ana I. Alfaro-Correa (Eds.). 1996. *Achieving Equitable Access: Studies of Health Care Issues Affecting Hispanics and African Americans*. Washington, DC: Joint Center for Political and Economic Studies Press. (Distributed by University Press of America, Lanham, MD.)

Link, Bruce, and Jo Phelan. 1995. "Social Conditions as Fundamental Causes of Disease." *Journal of Health and Social Behavior* 35 (Extra Issue): 80–94.

Link, Bruce G., and Jo C. Phelan. 2002. "McKeown and the Idea That Social Conditions Are Fundamental Causes of Disease." *American Journal of Public Health* 92: 730–732.

Liska, David. 1997. "Medicaid: Overview of a Complex Program." Publication No. A-8 in series Assessing New Federalism: Issues and Options for States. Washington, DC: The Urban Institute.

Long, Sharon K. 2003. "Hardship among the Uninsured: Choosing among Food, Housing, and Health Insurance." Publication No. B-54 in series New Federalism: National Survey of America's Families. Washington, DC: The Urban Institute.

Long, Sharon K., and Yu-Chu Shen. 2004. "Changing Options for Insurance Coverage: How Does the Future Look for Low- and Middle-Income Workers if Employer Sponsored Coverage Is Not an Option?" *Health Policy On-line*, No. 10. Washington, DC: The Urban Institute.

Loprest, Pamela. 2002. "Making the Transition from Welfare to Work: Successes but Continuing Concerns." In *Welfare Reform: The Next Act*, edited by Alan Weil and Kenneth Finegold, pp. 17–31. Washington, DC: The Urban Institute.

2003a. "Disconnected Welfare Leavers Face Serious Risk." Washington, DC: The Urban Institute.

2003b. "Fewer Welfare Leavers Employed in Weak Economy." Washington, DC: The Urban Institute.

Loury, Glenn C. 2001. "Politics, Race, and Poverty Research." In *Understanding Poverty*, edited by Sheldon H. Danziger and Robert H. Haveman. New York and Cambridge, MA: Russell Sage Foundation and Harvard University Press.

MacLanahan, Sara, and Gary Sandefur. 1994. *Growing Up with a Single Parent: What Hurts, What Helps*. Cambridge, MA: Harvard University Press.

Maioni, Antonia. 1998. *Parting at the Crossroads: The Emergence of Health Insurance in the United States and Canada*. Princeton, NJ: Princeton University Press.

Marmor, Theodore, and Morris L. Barer. 1997. "The Politics of Universal Health Insurance: Lessons from the 1990s." In *Health Politics and Policy*, edited by Theodor J. Litman and Leonard S. Robins, pp. 306–322. Washington, DC: Delmar Publishers.

Marmor, Theodore R. 1973. *The Politics of Medicare*. Chicago: Aldine.

Marmor, Theodore R., Jerry L. Mashaw, and Philip L. Harvey. 1990. *America's Misunderstood Welfare State: Persistent Myths, Enduring Realities*. New York: Basic Books.

Marshall, T. H. 1950. *Citizenship and Social Class, and Other Essays*. Cambridge: Cambridge University Press.

Massey, Douglas, and Nancy Denton. 1993. *American Apartheid*. Cambridge, MA: Harvard University Press.

McIntosh, Peggy. 1990. "White Privilege: Unpacking the Invisible Knapsack." *Independent School* 49: 31–35.

Mead, Lawrence M. 2001. "The Politics of Conservative Welfare Reform." In *The New World of Welfare*, edited by Rebecca M. Blank and Ron Haskins, pp. 201–220. Washington, DC: Brookings Institution Press.

Mills, Robert J., and Shailesh Bhandari. 2003. "Health Insurance Coverage in the United States: 2002." In *Current Population Reports*, pp. 60–223. Washington, DC: U.S. Bureau of the Census.

Mink, Gwendolyn. 1995. *The Wages of Motherhood: Inequality in the Welfare State, 1917–1942*. Ithaca, NY: Cornell University Press.

1998. *Welfare's End*. Ithaca, NY: Cornell University Press.

Moffitt, Robert. 1992. "Incentive Effects of the U.S. Welfare System: A Review." *Journal of Economic Literature* 30: 1–61.

2003a. "The Role of Non-financial Factors in Exit and Entry in the TANF Program." In *Welfare, Children, and Families*. Working Papers 03–02. Baltimore: Johns Hopkins University.

2003b. "The Temporary Assistance for Needy Families Program." In *Means-Tested Transfer Programs in the United States*, edited by Robert Moffitt, pp. 291–363. Chicago: University of Chicago Press.

Moffitt, Robert A. 2002. "From Welfare to Work: What the Evidence Shows," Policy Brief No. 13. In *Welfare Reform and Beyond*. Washington, DC: The Brookings Institution.

Moffitt, Robert, and Katie Winder. 2003. "The Correlates and Consequences of Welfare Exit and Entry: Evidence from the Three-City Study." Working Paper 03–01. Baltimore: Johns Hopkins University Press.

Moon, Marilyn. 1996. *Medicare Now and in the Future*. Washington, DC: The Urban Institute.

Morden, Nancy E., and Sean D. Sullivan. 2005. "States' Control of Prescription Drug Spending: A Heterogeneous Approach." *Health Affairs* 24: 1032–1038.

Mullahy, John, and Barbara Wolfe. 2001. "Health Policies for the Non-Elderly Poor." In *Understanding Poverty*, edited by Sheldon H. Danziger and Robert H. Haveman, pp. 278–313. New York and Cambridge, MA: Russell Sage Foundation and Harvard University Press.

Murdock, Steve H. 2004. "Slide 30: Population Change in Texas: Implications for Human and Socioeconomic Resources in the 21st Century." San Antonio: Texas State Data Center, The University of Texas at San Antonio.

Myles, John. 1989. *Old Age in the Welfare State: The Political Economy of Public Pensions*. Lawrence: University of Kansas Press.

National Association of Insurance Commissioners. 1999. "ERISA: Barrier to Health Care Consumers' Rights." Washington, DC: National Association of Insurance Commissioners.

Newman, Katherine S. 1999. *No Shame in My Game: The Working Poor in the Inner City*. New York: Alfred A. Knopf and the Russell Sage Foundation.

Newman, Katherine S. 2001. "Hard Times on 125th Street: Harlem's Poor Confront Welfare Reform." *American Anthropologist* 103: 762–778.

Noble, Charles. 1997. *Welfare as We Knew It: A Political History of the American Welfare State*. New York: Oxford University Press.

Numbers, Ronald L. 1978. *Almost Persuaded: American Physicians and Compulsory Health Insurance, 1912–1920*. Baltimore: Johns Hopkins University Press.

O'Connor, Alice. 2001. *Poverty Knowledge: Social Science, Social Policy, and the Poor in Twentieth-Century U.S. History*. Princeton, NJ: Princeton University Press.

Ogden, Cynthia L., Katherine M. Flegal, Margaret D. Carroll, and Clifford L. Johnson. 2002. "Prevalence and Trends in Overweight among US Children and Adolescents, 1999–2000." *Journal of the American Medical Association* 288: 1728–1732.

Pauly, Mark, and Bradley Herring. 2001. "Expanding Coverage via Tax Credits: Trade-offs and Outcomes." *Health Affairs* 20: 9–26.

Pepper Commission. 1990. "A Call for Action. Final Report to the U.S. Bipartisan Commission on Comprehensive Health Care." Washington, DC: U.S. Government Printing Office.

Perloff, Janet. 1999. "Insuring the Children: Obstacles and Opportunities." *Families in Society: The Journal of Contemporary Human Services* 80: 516–530.

Perry, Michael, Susan Kannel, R. Burciaga Valdez, and Christina Chang. 2000. "Medicaid and Children: Overcoming Barriers to Enrollment." Publication No. 2174. The Kaiser Commission on Medicaid and the Uninsured: Findings From a National Survey. Washington, DC: The Henry J. Kaiser Family Foundation.

Phillips, Shelly. 2003. "The Impact of Poverty on Health: A Scan of Research Literature." In *Canadian Population Health Initiative*, edited by Canadian Institute for Health Information. Ottawa: Canadian Institute for Health Information.

Phinney, Jean S. 1990. "Ethnic Identity in Adolescents and Adults: Review of Research." *Psychological Bulletin* 108: 499–514.

Pierson, Paul. 1994a. *Dismantling the Welfare State? Reagan, Thatcher, and the Politics of Retrenchment*. New York: Cambridge University Press.

1994b. "Increasing Returns: Path Dependence and the Study of Politics." *American Political Science Review* 94: 251–267.

2001a. "Coping with Permanent Austerity: Welfare State Restructuring in Affluent Democracies." In *The New Politics of the Welfare State*, edited by Paul Pierson, pp. 410–455. Oxford: Oxford University Press.

2001b. "Post-industrial Pressures on the Mature Welfare States." In *The New Politics of the Welfare State*, edited by Paul Pierson, pp. 80–106. Oxford: Oxford University Press.

Piven, Frances Fox. 1971. *Regulating the Poor: The Functions of Public Welfare*. New York: Pantheon Books.

Polivka, Anne, and Thomas Nardone. 1989. "On the Definition of 'Contingent Work.'" *Monthly Labor Review* 112: 9–16.

Portes, Alejandro, and Robert L. Bach. 1985. *Latin Journey: Cuban and Mexican Immigrants in the United States*. Berkeley: University of California Press.

Portes, Alejandro, and Rubén G. Rumbaut. 1997. *Immigrant America: A Portrait*. Los Angeles: University of California Press.

Quadagno, Jill. 1988a. "From Old-Age Assistance to Supplemental Security Income: The Political Economy of Relief in the South, 1935–1972." In *The Politics of Social Policy in the United States*, edited by Margaret Weir, Ann Shola Orloff, and Theda Skocpol. Princeton, NJ: Princeton University Press.

1988b. *The Transformation of Old Age Security: Class and Politics in the American Welfare State*. Chicago: University of Chicago Press.

1994. *The Color of Welfare: How Racism Undermined the War on Poverty.* New York: Oxford University Press.

2004. "Why the United States Has No National Health Insurance: Stakeholder Mobilization Against the Welfare State 1945–1996." *Journal of Health and Social Behavior* 45 (Extra Issue): 25–44.

2005. *One Nation, Uninsured: Why the U.S. Has No National Health Insurance.* New York: Oxford University Press.

Radzwill, M. 2003. "The Health Insurance Crisis in the United States: Lack of Access and the Ripple Effect." *Managed Care Interface* 16: 28–34.

Rank, Mark Robert. 1994. *Living on the Edge: The Realities of Welfare in America.* New York: Columbia University Press.

Reinhardt, Uwe E. 1998. "Employer-Based Health Insurance: R.I.P." In *The Future U.S. Healthcare System: Who Will Care for the Poor and Uninsured?*, edited by Stuart H. Altman, Uwe E. Reinhardt, and Alexandra E. Shields, pp. 325–352. Chicago: Health Administration Press.

Repetti, R. K., K. Matthews, and I. Waldron. 1989. "Employment and Women's Health: Effects of Paid Employment on Women's Mental and Physical Health." *American Psychologist* 44: 1394–1401.

Reschovsky, James D., and Peter J. Cunningham. 1998. "CHIPing Away at the Problem of Uninsured Children." Issue Brief No. 14. Washington, DC: Center for Studying Health System Change.

Rickelman, Bonnie L. 2002. "Demoralization as a Precursor to Serious Depression." *Journal of the American Psychiatric Nurses Association* 8: 9–19.

Robinson, James C. 2004. "Consolidation and the Transformation of Competition in Health Insurance." *Health Affairs* 23: 11–24.

Roetzheim, Richard G., Naazneen Pal, Eduardo C. Gonzalez, Jeanne M. Ferrante, Daniel J. Van Durme, and Jeffrey P. Krischer. 2000. "Effects of Health Insurance and Race on Colorectal Cancer Treatments and Outcomes." *American Journal of Public Health* 90: 1746–1754.

Rolett, Arlinda, Jennifer Parker, Katherine Heck, and Diane Makuc. 2001. "Parental Employment, Family Structure, and Child's Health Insurance." *Ambulatory Pediatrics* 1: 306–313.

Rosenau, Pauline Vaillancourt (Ed.). 2000. *Public-Private Policy Partnerships.* Cambridge, MA: The MIT Press.

Ross, Donna, and Laura Cox. 2000. "Making It Simple: Medicaid for Children and CHIP Income Eligibility Guidelines and Enrollment Procedures: Findings from a 50-State Survey." Washington, DC: Center for Budget and Policy Priorities.

Rowland, Diane, Alina Salganicoff, and Patricia Seliger Keenan. 1999. "The Key to the Door: Medicaid's Role in Improving Health Care for Women and Children." *Annual Review of Public Health* 20: 403–426.

Salganicoff, Alina, Usha R. Ranji, and Roberta Wyn. 2005. "Women and Health Care: A National Profile. Key Findings from the Kaiser Women's Health Survey." Washington, DC: The Henry J. Kaiser Family Foundation.

Salsberry, Pamela. 2003. "Why Are Some Children Still Uninsured?" *Journal of Pediatric Health Care* 17: 32–38.

Santos, R., and P. Seitz. 2000. "Benefit Coverage for Latino and Latina Workers." In *Moving Up the Economic Ladder: Latino Workers and the Nation's Future Prosperity*, edited by S. M. Perez, pp. 162–185. Washington, DC: National Council of La Raza.

Sawhill, Isabel V. 1995. "Welfare Reform: An Analysis of the Issues." Washington, DC: The Urban Institute.

Scarborough, Elinor. 2000. "West European Welfare States: The Old Politics of Retrenchment." *European Journal of Political Research* 38: 225–259.

Schexnayder, Deanna, Laura Lein, Karen Douglas, Daniel Shroeder, David Dominguez, and Freddie Richards. 2002. "Texas Families in Transition – Surviving Without TANF: An Analysis of Families Diverted from or Leaving TANF." Austin: Texas Department of Human Services.

Schlesinger, Arthur, Jr. 1992. *The Disuniting of America*. New York: Norton.

Schlesinger, Mark, and Karl Kronebusch. 1990. "The Failure of Parental Care Policy for the Poor." *Health Affairs* 9: 91–111.

Schoen, Cathy, Michelle M. Doty, Sara R. Collins, and Alyssa L. Holmgren. 2005. "Insured but Not Protected: How Many Adults Are Underinsured?" *Health Affairs*, 10.1377/hlthaff.w5.289 (June 14, 2005). *Web Exclusive*.

Schultze, Charles L. 2000. "Has Job Security Eroded for American Workers?" In *The New Relationship: Human Capital in the American Corporation*, edited by Margaret M. Blair and Thomas A. Kochan, pp. 28–65. Washington, DC: Brookings Institution Press.

Schur, C., L. Albers, and M. Berk 1995. "Health Care Use by Hispanic Adults: Financial vs. Non-financial Determinants." *Health Care Financing Review* 17: 71–88.

Sellers, Robert M., and J. Nicole Shelton. 2003. "The Role of Racial Identity in Perceived Racial Discrimination." *Journal of Personality and Social Psychology* 84: 1079–1092.

Shaffer, Ellen R. 2003. "Universal Coverage and Public Health: New State Studies." *American Journal of Public Health* 93: 109–111.

Shah-Canning, D., J. J. Alpert, and H. Bauchner. 1996. "Care-Seeking Patterns of Inner-City Families Using an Emergency Room. A Three-Decade Comparison." *Medical Care* 34: 1171–1179.

Shapiro, Thomas M. 2003. *The Hidden Cost of Being African American: How Wealth Perpetuates Inequality*. New York: Oxford University Press.

Shen, Yu-Chu, and Steven Zuckerman. 2003. "Why Is There State Variation in Employer-Sponsored Insurance?" *Health Affairs* 22: 241–251.

Singer, Burton H., and Carol D. Ryff (Eds.). 2001. *New Horizons in Health: An Integrative Approach*. Washington, DC: National Academy Press.

Skocpol, Theda. 1996. *Boomerang: Clinton's Health Security Effort and the Turn Against Government in U.S. Politics*. New York: Norton.

Smeeding, Timothy M. 2000. "Changing Income Inequality in OECD Countries: Updated Results from the Luxembourg Income Study (LIS)." In *The Personal Distribution of Income in an International Perspective*, edited by Richard Hauser and Irene Becker, pp. 205–224. Berlin: Springer-Verlag.

Smeeding, Timothy M., Lee Rainwater, and Gary Burtless. 2001. "U.S. Poverty in a Cross-National Context." In *Understanding Poverty*, edited by Sheldon H. Danziger and Robert H. Haveman, pp. 162–89. New York and Cambridge, MA: Russell Sage Foundation and Harvard University Press.

Smith, Vernon K., and David M. Rousseau. 2003. "SCHIP Program Enrollment: June 2003 Update." Publication No. 4148. The Kaiser Commission on Medicaid and the Uninsured. Washington, DC: The Henry J. Kaiser Family Foundation.

Smith, Vernon K., David M. Rousseau, and Molly O'Malley. 2004. "SCHIP Program Enrollment: December 2003 Update." Publication No. 7134. The Kaiser Commission on Medicaid and the Uninsured. Washington, DC: The Henry J. Kaiser Family Foundation.

Smith, Vernon, Rekha Ramesh, Kathleen Gifford, Eileen Ellis, Victoria Wachino, and Molly O'Malley. 2004. "States Respond to Fiscal Pressure: A 50-State Update of State Medicaid Spending Growth and Cost Containment Actions." Report (#0000). The Kaiser Commission on Medicaid and the Uninsured. Washington, DC: The Henry J. Kaiser Family Foundation. URL: http://kff.org/medicaid/loader.cfm?url=/commonspot/security/getfile.cfm&PageID=30453. Accessed February 14, 2006.

Social Security Administration. 2004a. "The 2004 Annual Report of the Board of Trustees of the Federal Old-Age and Survivors Insurance and Disability Insurance Trust Fund." Table IV.B2. Washington, DC: Social Security Administration.

———. 2004b. "Ratio of Social Security Covered Workers to Beneficiaries Calendar Years: 1940–2000." Washington, DC: Social Security Administration.

Spalter-Roth, Roberta, and Heidi Hartmann. 1998. "Gauging the Consequences for Gender Relations, Pay Equity, and the Public Purse." In *Contingent Work: American Employment Relations in Transition*, edited by Kathleen Barker and Kathleen Christensen, pp. 69–100. Ithaca, NY: Cornell University Press.

Sparer, Michael S. 2000. "Myths and Misunderstandings." In *Public–Private Policy Partnerships*, edited by Pauline Villancourt Rosenau, pp. 143–159. Cambridge, MA: The MIT Press.

Stack, Carol. 1997. *All Our Kin*. New York: Basic Books.

Starfield, Barbara. 2000. "Evaluating the State Children's Health Insurance Program: Critical Considerations." *Annual Review of Public Health* 21: 569–585.

Starr, Paul. 1982. *The Social Transformation of American Medicine*. New York: Basic Books.

1994. *The Logic of Health Care Reform: Why and How the President's Plan Will Work*. New York: Whittle Books, in association with Penguin Books.

Stephens, John D. 1996. "The Scandinavian Welfare States: Achievements, Crisis, and Prospects." In *Welfare States in Transition: National Adaptations in Global Economies*, edited by Gøsta Esping-Andersen, pp. 32–65. London: Sage.

Stephens, John D., Evelyne Huber, and Leonard Ray. 1999. "The Welfare State in Hard Times." In *Continuity and Change in Contemporary Capitalism*, edited by Herbert Kitschelt, Peter Lange, Gary Marks, and John D. Stephens, pp. 164–193. Cambridge: Cambridge University Press.

Stern, M. P., M. Rosenthal, S. M. Haffner, H. P. Hazuda, and L. J. Franco. 1984. "Sex Difference in the Effects of Sociocultural Status on Diabetes and Cardiovascular Risk Factors in Mexican Americans: The San Antonio Heart Study." *American Journal of Epidemiology* 120: 834–851.

Stern, Michael P., Clicerio Gonzalez, Braxton D. Mitchell, Enrique Villalpando, Steven M. Haffner, and Helen P. Hazuda. 1992. "Genetic and Environmental Determinants of Type II Diabetes in Mexico City and San Antonio." *Diabetes* 41: 489–492.

Stevens, Beth. 1988. "Blurring the Boundaries: How the Federal Government Has Influenced Welfare Benefits in the Private Sector." In *The Politics of Social Policy in the United States*, edited by Margaret Weir, Ann Shola Orloff, and Theda Skocpol, pp. 123–148. Princeton, NJ: Princeton University Press.

Strayhorn, Carole Keeyon. 2001. "Section I: Medicaid Program." In *Texas Health Care Claims Study*. Texas Comptroller of Public Accounts, Austin: Texas Office of the Comptroller.

Sullivan, Teresa A., Elizabeth Warren, and Jay Lawrence Westbrook. 2000. *Fragile Middle Class: Americans in Debt*. New Haven, CT: Yale University Press.

Sumner, William Graham. 1883. *What Social Classes Owe Each Other*. New York: Harper and Brothers.

Suro, Roberto. 1998. *Strangers among Us: How Latino Immigration Is Transforming America*. New York: Alfred A. Knopf.

Suro, Roberto, and Audrey Singer. 2002. "Latino Growth in Metropolitan America: Changing Patterns, New Locations." Washington, DC: The Brookings Institution.

Swank, Duane. 2001. "Political Institutions and Welfare State Restructuring: The Impact of Institutions on Social Policy Change in Developed Democracies." In *The New Politics of the Welfare State*, edited by Paul Pierson, pp. 197–237. Oxford: Oxford University Press.

Taylor, J. Edward, Philip E. Martin, and Michael Fix. 1997. *Poverty Amid Prosperity: Immigration and the Changing Face of Rural California.* Washington, DC: Urban Institute Press.

Teles, Steven Michael. 1996. *Whose Welfare? AFDC and Elite Politics.* Lawrence: University of Kansas Press.

Thamer, Mae, and Christian Richard. 1997. "Health Insurance Coverage among Foreign-Born US Residents: The Impact of Race, Ethnicity, and Length of Residence." *American Journal of Public Health* 87: 96–102.

Thompson, Allison. 1999. "Industry Output and Employment Projections to 2008." *Monthly Labor Review* 122: 33–50.

Thompson, Karen MacDonald, and Doris F. Glick. 1999. "Cost Analysis of Emergency Room Use by Low-Income Patients." *Nursing Economics* 17: 142–148.

Tilly, Chris. 2004. "Raw Deal for Workers: Why Have U.S. Workers Experienced a Long-Term Decline in Pay, Benefits, and Working Conditions?" *International Journal of Health Services* 34: 305–311.

Tooker, John. 2002. "Affordable Health Insurance for All Is Possible by Means of a Pragmatic Approach." *American Journal of Public Health* 93: 106–109.

Tumlin, Karen, Wendy Zimmerman, and Jason Ost. 1999. "State Snapshots of Public Benefits for Immigrants: A Supplement Report to 'Patchwork Policies.'" Occasional Paper 24 in series Assessing the New Federalism. New York: The Urban Institute.

U.S. Bureau of the Census. 1998. "Measuring 50 Years of Economic Change Using the March Current Population Survey." In *Current Population Reports,* series P60-203. Washington, DC: U.S. Government Printing Office.

2000. "Percent of Persons Who Are Asian Alone: 2000." TM-P004D. *American Fact Finder.* Washington, DC: U.S. Bureau of the Census.

2003a. "Children's Living Arrangements and Characteristics: March 2002." In *Current Population Reports,* series P20–547. Washington, DC: U.S. Government Printing Office.

2003b. "Cities with 250,000 or More Inhabitants in 2000 – Hispanic and Non-Hispanic Groups: 2000." Table No. 32. In *Statistical Abstract of the United States: 2003,* p. 399. Washington, DC: U.S. Bureau of the Census.

U.S. Census Bureau. 2005. "Income Stable, Poverty Up, Numbers of Americans with and without Health Insurance Rise." *International Journal of Health Services* 35: 117–124.

U.S. Department of Health and Human Services. 2000. *Healthy People 2010, Understanding and Improving Health,* 2nd edition. 2 vols. Washington, DC: U.S. Government Printing Office.

U.S. Department of Justice. 2005. "Introduction to Federal Voting Rights Laws: The Voting Rights Act of 1965." Washington, DC: U.S. Department of Justice.

Valdez, R. B., A. Giachello, H. Rodrigues-Trias, P. Gomez, and C. de la Rocha. 1993. "Access to Health Care in Latino Communities." *Public Health Reports* 108: 534–549.

Vastag, Brian. 2002. "Education Needed to Expand SCHIP Eligibility." *Journal of the American Medical Association* 287: 1101.

Vinicor, F. 1994. "Is Diabetes a Public-Health Disorder?" *Diabetes Care* 17 (Supplement 1): 22–27.

Weil, Alan. 2001. "Increments toward What? Incremental Steps Taken Today Affect the Options Available for Future Coverage Expansions." *Health Affairs* 20: 68–82.

Weinick, Robin, and Nancy Krauss. 2000. "Racial/Ethnic Differences in Children's Access to Care." *American Journal of Public Health* 90: 1771–1774.

Weir, Margaret, Ann Shola Orloff, and Theda Skocpol. 1988. *The Politics of Social Policy in the United States*. Princeton, NJ: Princeton University Press.

Welch, Finis. 1999. "In Defense of Inequality." *The American Economic Review* 89: 1–17.

Weller, Christian E., Jeffrey Wenger, and Elise Gould. 2004. *Health Insurance Coverage in Retirement: The Erosion of Retiree Income Security*. Washington, DC: Economic Policy Institute.

Wheaton, Laura. 1998. "Low-Income Families and the Marriage Tax." In *Strengthening Families*, Number 1. Washington, DC: The Urban Institute.

Wicks, Elliot K. 2003. "Issues in Expansion Coverage Design: Decision Points and Trade-offs in Developing Comprehensive Health Coverage Reforms." In *Covering America: Real Remedies for the Uninsured*. Washington, DC: Economic and Social Research Institute.

Wielawski, Irene. 2000. "Gouging the Medically Uninsured: A Tale of Two Bills." *Health Affairs* 19: 180–185.

Williams, Claudia, James Rosen, Julie Hudman, and Molly O'Malley. 2004. "Challenges and Trade-offs in Low-Income Family Budgets: Implications for Health Coverage." Publication No. 4147. The Kaiser Commission on Medicaid and the Uninsured. Washington, DC: The Henry J. Kaiser Family Foundation.

Williams, David R., and Chiquita Collins. 1995. "U.S. Socioeconomic and Racial Differences in Health Patterns and Explanations." *Annual Review of Sociology* 29: 349–386.

Wilson, William J. 1978. *The Declining Significance of Race: Blacks and Changing American Institutions*. Chicago: University of Chicago Press.

1987. *The Truly Disadvantaged: The Inner City, the Underclass, and Public Policy*. Chicago: University of Chicago Press.

Wilson, William Julius. 1999. *The Bridge over the Racial Divide: Rising Inequality and Coalition Politics*. Berkeley: University of California Press.

Winkleby, M. A., and C. Cubbins. 2003. "Influence of Individual and Neighborhood Socioeconomic Status on Mortality among Black,

Mexican-American, and White Women and Men in the United States." *Journal of Epidemiology and Community Health* 57: 444–452.

Winston, Pamela, Ronald J. Angel, Linda M. Burton, P. Lindsay Chase-Lansdale, Andrew J. Cherlin, Robert A. Moffitt, and William. J. Wilson. 1999. *Welfare, Children and Families: Overview and Design.* Baltimore: Johns Hopkins University Press.

Wolfe, Barbara, and David Vanness. 1999. "Inequality in Health Care Access and Utilization and the Potential Role for the Public Sector." In *Fighting Poverty: Caring for Children, Parents, the Elderly, and Health*, edited by Stein Ringen and Philip R. de Jong, pp. 251–286. Brookfield, MA: Aldershot.

Wu, Jasmanda H., Mary N. Haan, Jersey Liang, Debashis Ghosh, Hector M. Gonzalez, and William H. Herman. 2003. "Diabetes as a Predictor of Change in Functional Status among Older Mexican Americans: A Population-Based Cohort Study." *Diabetes Care* 26: 314–319.

Zambrana, Ruth E., and Laura A. Logie. 2000. "Latino Child Health: Need for Inclusion in the U.S. National Discourse." *American Journal of Public Health* 90: 1827–1833.

Zimmerman, Wendy, and Karen Tumlin. 1999. "Patchwork Policies: State Assistance for Immigrants under Welfare Reform." Occasional Papers. Washington, DC: The Urban Institute.

Zuckerman, Stephen, Genevieve Kenney, Lisa Dubay, Jennifer Haley, and John Holahan. 2001. "Shifting Health Insurance Coverage, 1997–1999: Economic Expansion, Welfare Reform, and SCHIP Have Changed Who Has Insurance Coverage, but not Across the Board." *Health Affairs* 20: 169–177.

Zweifel, Peter, and Willard G. Manning. 2000. "Moral Hazard and Consumer Incentives in Health Care." In *Handbook of Health Economics,* volume 1A, edited by Anthony J. Culyer and Joseph Newhouse, pp. 410–459. Amsterdam: Elsevier.

Index

AARP (American Association of
Retired Persons), 196–197
ADHD (attention deficit
hyperactivity disorder), 164
AFDC, failure of, 27
African Americans
in Boston, 81–82, 87, 130, 132
Cecilia's case, 1–5
in Chicago, 80, 87, 130, 132
Claudia's case, 146–148
Darlene's case, 64, 67
and demoralization, 137–143
discrimination and racism against,
24–25, 44–45, 130, 132, 134
education of, 183
employment of, 22, 36, 183
health care coverage for, 172, 182
and immunization of children, 192
and obesity of children, 192–193
on racial and ethnic tensions, 155
and rejection of racial or ethnic
attribution for problems, 139
residential exclusion and
segregation of, 131–132,
136–137, 147, 148–149
in San Antonio, 87, 130, 132, 156
Sarah's case, 33–34
Sonia's case, 101–105, 114–116,
123–124, 143–146

statistics on child poverty, 23–24
in Three City Study, 8–9
and uninsured children, 93
vulnerability, health and,
132–136
in workforce of future, 48,
210–211
see also race and ethnicity
aging, see elderly
AIDS/HIV, 41, 141, 168
allergies, 19
American Association of Retired
Persons (AARP), 196–197
American Medical Association, 46
Anita, 64, 70–72
child of, 71
dental care for, 72
employment of, 71
health problems of, 71
in job training and placement
program, 71
and Medicaid, 64, 71–72
medical debt of, 70–72
Temporary Assistance to Needy
Families (TANF) for, 71
Arrow, Kenneth, 197, 198
Asians, 87
asthma, 19, 33–34, 73, 103, 117,
164, 179